Lose Weight, Gain Ene

date shown.

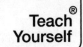

Lose Weight, Gain Energy, Get Healthy

Sara Kirkham

For UK order enquiries: please contact Bookpoint Ltd,
130 Milton Park, Abingdon, Oxon OX14 4SB.
Telephone: +44 (0) 1235 827720. Fax: +44 (0) 1235 400454.
Lines are open 09.00–17.00, Monday to Saturday, with a 24-hour
message answering service. Details about our titles and how to
order are available at www.teachyourself.com

Long renowned as the authoritative source for self-guided learning –
with more than 50 million copies sold worldwide – the **Teach Yourself**
series includes over 500 titles in the fields of languages, crafts, hobbies,
business, computing and education.

British Library Cataloguing in Publication Data: a catalogue record
for this title is available from the British Library.

First published in UK 2007 by Hodder Education,
338 Euston Road, London, NW1 3BH

This edition published 2010.

Previously published as *Teach Yourself Eating for Health*.

The **Teach Yourself** name is a registered trade mark of
Hodder Headline.

Typeset by MPS Limited, A Macmillan Company.

Printed in Great Britain for Hodder Education, an Hachette
UK Company, 338 Euston Road, London NW1 3BH, by
CPI Cox & Wyman, Reading, Berkshire RG1 8EX.

The publisher has used its best endeavours to ensure that the URLs
for external websites referred to in this book are correct and active
at the time of going to press. However, the publisher and the
author have no responsibility for the websites and can make no
guarantee that a site will remain live or that the content will remain
relevant, decent or appropriate.

Hachette UK's policy is to use papers that are natural, renewable
and recyclable products and made from wood grown in sustainable
forests. The logging and manufacturing processes are expected to
conform to the environmental regulations of the country of origin.

Impression number   10 9 8 7 6 5 4 3 2 1
Year   2014 2013 2012 2011 2010

Acknowledgements

For my mum and dad, who must have instilled some healthy eating habits into me early on, in addition to giving me the drive to follow my dreams in life and do what I want to do.

For my husband Keith who, luckily for me, enjoys rather than endures our healthy eating regimen at home, and motivates me to eat healthily (most of the time!) almost as much as I do him.

For all of our family and friends who have accommodated my dietary preferences on many enjoyable occasions at their homes.

For the 'tea break crew' for proofreading some of the chapters for me.

For everyone who has enabled and supported my quest to know more about nutrition and make it my vocation in life, through either playing a part in my endless years of study or by providing the opportunities for me to share this knowledge and passion with others.

Contents

Meet the author   xi
Only got a minute?   xii
Only got five minutes?   xiv
Only got ten minutes?   xvi

1 Food for health and life   1
   What is a healthy diet?   2
   Your food diary   2
   Healthy eating recommendations   4
   Optimum nutrition   14
   Nutrition quiz   16
   Understanding the basics   20
   Proof that a healthy diet works   26

2 Eat to lose weight   29
   Reasons for weight gain   29
   The Energy Balance Equation   30
   Calculating your Body Mass Index   32
   Basal Metabolic Rate   35
   How much weight should you lose?   36
   1 Reducing your calorie intake   40
   2 Using up more calories through activity and exercise   50
   3 Eating less and exercising more   54
   Seven-day eating plan for healthy weight loss   55

3 Superfoods   60
   What are superfoods?   61
   Phytonutrients   61
   The essential fatty acids   66
   Meet the superfoods   69
   Simple tips for increasing your superfood intake   78
   Superfoods seven-day eating plan   82
   Superfood recipes   84
   Getting the most from superfoods   89

4 How to detox!   92
   Why detox?   93
   Do YOU need to detox?   95

What are toxins? 96
How we detoxify 97
Detox options 100
Planning your detox 104
Top ten foods for detox 107
Basic detox guidelines 108
Supplements to help 110
What to expect during your detox 112
Possible side effects 113
Fourteen-day detox eating plan 117

5 Functional foods 123
What are functional foods? 124
Are functional foods useful? 127
Benefits and drawbacks of functional foods 128
Omega 3 fatty acids 130
Plant sterols 137
Do functional foods cost more? 141
The probiotic and prebiotic revolution 142
Will functional foods work for you? 147

6 How to look (and be!) younger 151
What is ageing? 152
Top ten anti-ageing diet tips 155
Anti-ageing nutrients 168
Nutrition for super skin 173
Water 176
Does diet affect your hair and nails? 177
Your anti-ageing guide 179

7 Energy boosting foods 185
Where do we get energy from? 186
Glycaemic Index (GI) and Glycaemic Load (GL) 187
Blood sugar control 189
How much carbohydrate should you eat? 193
Energy giving foods 193
Water 195
Caffeinated drinks 197
Stress 199
Adrenal superfoods 199
Health conditions that can sap vitality 200

8   **Food for thought**   **214**
    Serotonin   215
    Chocolate – friend or foe?   216
    Brain food – fish and fish oils   219
    Nutrients for brain power   224
    The effect of low blood sugar levels   229
    Dietary benefits for specific mental health conditions   230
    Supplements to help mental function   244
9   **Healthy eating for the family**   **249**
    Small steps   250
    Healthy meal ideas   251
    Cutting a few corners!   258
    Get the family involved   260
    Going organic   264
    Grow your own   267
    Taking it further   **271**
      Further reading   **271**
      Useful websites   **272**
    Index   **274**

Meet the author

Welcome to *Lose Weight, Gain Energy, Get Healthy*!

Hello! I hope that you will find this book inspirational and informative, and perhaps make it your personal nutrition guide! My aim was to write a book based upon factual nutritional information, encompassing every tool and tip I have come across and used in the past 20 years to help people eat a healthier diet. I find that many people have a good idea about what they should be eating for health, but find it difficult to put it into practice. Therefore, you won't find a bible of optimum nutrition here, telling you what you should and shouldn't eat, but you will find all the facts you need to create a healthy, balanced diet, and make those all-important changes.

In each chapter I have addressed an important aspect of diet and health, though much of my dietary advice crops up in more than one chapter – proof that making just one dietary change can have several different health benefits. Specific health-promoting properties of particular foods are also employed, with diets to help reduce cholesterol, beautify skin, and manage inflammatory diseases such as arthritis or eczema.

My hope is that by using this interactive, information guide as your personal nutrition guide you can make the journey towards a healthier diet and a healthier you! Once you have digested one chapter, you're sure to be back for a second helping – healthy eating has never tasted so good, nor been so easy!

Only got a minute?

You have no doubt heard the expression 'You are what you eat', and this is absolutely true – every cell in our body is formed from the nutrients we take in as food, so what you eat has a direct effect upon your health, and how you look and feel. You can make no better change for yourself or your family than to eat a healthier diet, and despite the wealth of conflicting information out there, there are many simple and proven dietary fundamentals that are known to enhance good health. For example, we know that we need a varied diet containing all the food groups, vitamins and minerals for continued health, and we need to balance our energy (calorie) intake with our expenditure in order to maintain a healthy weight. However, there are so many other advantages gained from following a healthy diet...

> ► Enhanced energy levels
> ► Radiant skin
> ► Improved ability to cope with stress

- ► Better sleep
- ► Lower blood pressure
- ► Lower cholesterol levels
- ► Stronger bones
- ► Better digestion
- ► Reduced risk of some cancers

... and these are just a few of the benefits. Positive results attributable to healthy eating encompass body size and shape, disease prevention and mood enhancement. If you know someone who looks much younger than they actually are, what and how they eat is likely to have contributed to this enigma.

Getting started is simple – all you need is a credible source of information combined with lots of practical tips, and of course, shopping lists, recipes and eating plans all help to make healthy eating an enjoyable part of your life rather than yet another 'diet'. A good way to start is to go food shopping for all the healthy foods you need for the week – healthy eating is much easier with a kitchen full of nutritious foods, and it should become a way of life, not a diet... so what are you waiting for?

5 Only got five minutes?

By following a nutritious and balanced diet you are guaranteed to look and feel better, and your health will also benefit. Several large-scale studies suggest a positive association between fruit and vegetable consumption, and decreased risk of heart disease and various cancers – you can reduce your risk of heart disease by 4 per cent for each additional portion of vegetables, and by 7 per cent for each additional portion of fruit eaten! So whether you want to lose weight or just eat a healthy diet, fruit and vegetables should always form a significant part of your food intake. Of course we need other types of food for good health as well: starchy carbohydrates such as rice, oats or potatoes provide a more concentrated source of energy than fruits and vegetables and we also need foods containing protein and fats to provide a full range of essential nutrients.

Because each food group provides different nutrients and has different roles in the body, it's never a good idea to omit any food group from your diet completely. You can choose to reduce the amount of fat in your diet if you want to reduce calorie and/ or fat intake, but we must take in the essential fatty acids (found in fish, nuts, seeds and vegetable oils) and ensure that we are getting enough of the fat soluble vitamins A, D, E and K. Limiting carbohydrate intake has been a popular diet to follow, but we do need carbohydrate foods for energy and to supply a range of vitamins, minerals and phytonutrients.

In short, if a 'diet' cannot be followed long term for any reason, particularly health issues, then you should re-consider whether you should follow it at all. Any quick gains are short lived because once you return to your normal diet you will find you have not changed your 'normal' eating habits, and will quickly be back where you started! Making slow but sure improvements to your existing diet is a more effective way of reaching your goals in the long run.

You should aim to increase rather than decrease the range of foods that you eat, creating an eating habit that you can enjoy and sustain for life.

However, although most of us already have an idea of what we should be eating for good health, actually doing it is often more difficult. Putting a new eating regime into practice can be a big change, but with practical tips and recipes to help, healthy eating is much easier and enjoyable. Even challenging situations like losing weight or cooking for the family are possible with a plethora of helpful tips and a toolbox of tricks. Changing your eating habits can mean a big adjustment in lifestyle, and it can be tough (which is why so many diets fail), but the trick is to make small changes, take tiny steps rather than big leaps, and give yourself (and your family) time to get used to each new change before you introduce another one. Taking small steps towards a healthier diet and maintaining each change will eventually get you to where you want to be, whereas trying to follow an 'optimum nutrition' diet usually lasts for about three days before you fall back into your old eating habits. Deciding where you are now, what you want to achieve, and planning the changes you aim to make, are all important elements of lifestyle change, and will get you off to a good start. However, to stick with your new eating plan, it has to be enjoyable, or it won't last. Take a look at these tips to help you create a diet that you actually want to follow!

- ▶ Eating fruit doesn't have to be boring. Make up a colourful fruit salad so it's ready to eat and you're much more likely to choose this for breakfast/snacks/dessert than pick up an apple out of the fruit bowl! Try different types of melon mixed with berries, kiwi, pineapple and red grapes.
- ▶ Buy or prepare vegetable crudités so these are ready to eat and more likely to tempt you away from the biscuit barrel. Have healthy dips like hummus to dip your veggie sticks into for additional flavour. Try strips of pepper, baby sweetcorn, mange tout, asparagus spears – it doesn't have to be celery and carrot sticks!

10 Only got ten minutes?

With what appears to be conflicting advice and different types of diets constantly being promoted, eating a healthy diet may not seem that straight forward! That's why it is so important to take your inspiration from educated and well researched dietary sources, and avoid the latest diet craze, even (and especially) if it does promise incredible weight loss or extraordinary health results. The principles of a healthy diet are really quite straight forward and, when followed, will have a significant beneficial effect upon the way that you look and feel. The basic principles of a healthy balanced diet are as follows:

1 Base your meals on starchy foods.
2 Eat lots of fruit and vegetables.
3 Eat more fish.
4 Cut down on saturated fat and sugar.
5 Try to eat less salt – no more than 6 g a day.
6 Get active and try to be a healthy weight.
7 Drink plenty of water.
8 Don't skip breakfast.

Simple! But if you are looking for a little more inspiration rather than information, there is a plethora of research regarding the benefits of the so-called Mediterranean diet that is known to promote better health. Individual aspects of this dietary approach each hold their own merits. Increased fish consumption boosts our omega-3 intake which can promote better mental function and reduce inflammatory conditions; olive oil has known cardio-protective and anti-fungal properties; and consuming more natural foods such as nuts, fruits and vegetables boosts nutrient intake and improves health in a number of different ways, so these are good foods upon which to base your diet. The benefits of a diet like this are that the whole family can eat in this way and expect to improve their health as a result. Of course, if everyone in the household is eating the same foods, this makes for a much easier life as well!

In addition to creating a basic healthy diet, you can adapt your individual eating plan further to suit yourself and to enable you to achieve your personal goals, whether that might be weight loss, more energy, or better skin. Adapting your diet in this way creates a basic healthy diet platform from which you can manipulate and individualize your diet to suit you.

1 *Make sure your diet contains all the food groups (carbohydrates, proteins and fats) and is made up of predominantly fresh, un-processed produce.*
2 *Include foods and preparation methods known to be healthy, such as those of the Mediterranean diet – eat plenty of vegetables, fruit and fish, and swap some of the saturated fats found in meat and dairy for polyunsaturated fats found in fish and vegetable oils.*
3 *Now personalize your diet to suit you – add superfoods for better health or for specific benefits such as better skin, more energy or improved mental function.*

Here are some more ideas to make healthy eating easier; hopefully you'll be inspired to create a superfood diet that will enable you to achieve your dietary and health goals.

▶ To aid weight loss and improve health, swap normal potatoes for sweet potatoes – more nutrients, less calories! As well as containing fewer calories than a normal potato; the beta carotene levels in sweet potatoes also boost your anti-oxidant intake, support immune function and aid natural detoxification. If you prefer to follow a diet lower in starch (complex carbohydrates), this could also be a useful alternative to satisfy those potato cravings!
▶ If weight loss is your goal, try eating slowly and reducing your portion sizes. Just making these two changes can reduce your food and calorie intake, without actually making any changes to the types of food that you eat.
▶ Your first step towards a superfood diet is to increase your nutrient intake – for instance, swap cos or iceberg lettuce for

dark green spinach, rocket or watercress which all contain higher levels of calcium, magnesium, iron and vitamin C.

▶ For a DIY mini-detox, start each day with a glass of hot water with a slice of lemon or lime. The hot water is too warm to be absorbed through the stomach or small intestine, so it travels on to the large intestine (bowel) and helps to dislodge material adhering to the bowel wall. The additional water also helps to bulk out the stool and allow easier peristalsis along the bowel.

▶ Rather than rely on expensive functional foods to lower your cholesterol levels, include garlic, onion, chicory, Jerusalem artichokes and asparagus in your diet. These foods contain a fibre called inulin which absorbs cholesterol and carries it out of the body when the fibre is eliminated via the bowel.

▶ Some nutrients have specific health benefits. Take, for example, Brazil nuts – because of their selenium content they make a great anti-ageing anti-oxidant 'supplement'! In fact, most nuts contain helpful levels of anti-oxidants Vitamin E, selenium and zinc... all contributing to better skin health too.

▶ Research shows that of all the things we ask for, 'more energy' is one of the most common requests, yet this can be one of the quickest and easiest things to correct in our diet, as being just 4 per cent dehydrated can reduce our energy levels by up to 25 per cent! Make sure you drink eight glasses of water a day to feel energized and full of get up and go.

▶ Swapping two meals a week from meat to fish can improve allergies and inflammatory skin conditions and boost mental function, as well as delivering the healthy benefits of the Mediterranean diet to your heart.

▶ If lack of time is your barrier to healthy eating, an extra baked potato or additional rice portion cooked for dinner can provide the beginnings of potato or cold rice salad for tomorrow's healthy lunch – it takes no extra time, and can provide the healthy tuck box lunches you and your family have been looking for.

Although a strong connection between food and wellbeing has existed for centuries, we are only just beginning to understand the association between our diet and health. For example, ground-breaking research is now illustrating important links between fatty acid deficiency and impaired cognitive function, or conditions such as dementia, depression and attention deficit hyperactivity disorder. Whether your aspiration is to look or feel better, you will find no better way than a healthy diet to help you achieve your goal. So why don't you start on your journey towards a healthier diet and a healthier you right now... you'll never look back!

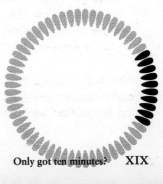

1

Food for health and life

In this chapter you will learn:
* *how to keep a food diary*
* *how to eat a healthy, balanced diet*
* *how good or bad your current diet is.*

In AD390 Hippocrates said 'Let food be your medicine and medicine be your food', and people have used the properties and nutrients in foods since that time. For example, in herbal medicine, apples have often been used to help prevent or reduce constipation, prompting the saying 'An apple a day keeps the doctor away'. Blueberries were historically used to alleviate food poisoning or diarrhoea, and we now know that these berries contain anti-bacterial compounds that help to fight gastrointestinal infections.

You can be your own food doctor – supporting your health and improving the way you look and feel by adjusting your diet to suit your needs. Whether you want to lose weight, look younger, or improve your health, you can have a positive effect upon your health by changing the foods that you eat. What could be better than finding an easy and inexpensive way to feel healthy and look great? The answer we're all looking for is right in front of us, in the foods that we eat every day. You have a food pharmacy at your fingertips, right there in your kitchen!

Case study

After repeated gastrointestinal problems owing to a poor diet with little fibre, Amy was due to have surgery on her bowel. In desperation, she sought help from a nutritionist to change her diet, and after just three weeks of following the diet, her bowel was working perfectly and there was no need for an operation. Needless to say, she stopped 'living' on chocolate and continued with a healthy, high fibre diet after that!

What is a healthy diet?

With so much conflicting information on what we should and shouldn't eat, it's no surprise that so many people are confused about what a healthy diet really is! In addition to Health Authority recommendations, there are guidelines from organizations such as the British Heart Foundation, World Health Organization and Food Standards Agency, hundreds of diet books and fad diets in every magazine you pick up, and on top of this we are bombarded with food industry promotions for functional foods, low GI products, foods that are low in sugar, reduced salt, low fat or organic. Which sources of information can you trust?

Your food diary

A good place to start is to create to a list of the foods you eat each day – this is known as a food diary – and assess it. Ask yourself the following questions and add up how much of each type of food you ate at the bottom of your food diary – the numbers of servings you ideally want to consume are shown in brackets after each food group:

How many meals were based upon starchy carbohydrates? (3)
How many servings of fruit and vegetables were eaten? (5+)
How many servings of dairy foods were eaten? (2–3)

How many servings of protein foods were eaten? (2–3)
How many fatty or sugary foods were eaten? (minimum)

Your food diary might look like this:

Food diary

	MONDAY	TUESDAY	WEDNESDAY
Breakfast	Cornflakes with sugar, skimmed milk and a banana Cup of black coffee	Porridge with soya milk and berries Cup of black coffee	2 slices of toast with butter and jam Mug of tea – milk, 2 sugars
Lunch	Tuna mayonnaise salad sandwich and juice	Baked potato with cheese and juice	Ham sandwich (with butter) and cup of tea (as above)
Dinner	Spaghetti bolognaise with cheese topping Glass of wine	Salmon steak, broccoli and carrots	Beans on toast Mug of tea (as above)
Snacks	Apple	Yoghurt	–
Drinks	2 glasses of water	2 cups of tea, 2 sugars	2 glasses of water
Guidelines			
Starchy foods (3)	3	2	3
Fruit and veg (5)	4	4	1
Dairy foods (2–3)	2	2	2
Protein foods (2–3)	2	2	2
Sugars and fats	3	3	5

This is a simple, but illustrative guide to knowing whether your diet is healthy and balanced. Straight away you can see whether you're eating enough fruit and vegetables, or consuming too much dairy produce, for example. This then provides you with a way of monitoring your progress as you adjust your diet – you can choose something to concentrate on, such as increasing your fruit and vegetable intake, and add up the portions you eat every day.

There are several additional benefits of keeping a food diary:

✓ *You can also monitor your water intake, aiming for eight glasses a day.*
✓ *You can monitor your intake of coffee and alcohol.*
✓ *You can add how you're feeling after each meal (a food and mood diary) – this helps you to pinpoint foods that might not suit you.*
✓ *Keeping a food diary also makes you more aware of what you are (and aren't) eating, and often prompts healthier eating habits.*
✓ *It can also help with weight loss (see Chapter 2 for further advice on how to use your food diary in this way).*

Healthy eating recommendations

It is worth bearing in mind that food manufacturers will always want to sell their product, and whilst the information provided should be correct, it may be biased. Avoid fad diets that seem to cut out entire foods or food groups, or promise results that seem too good to be true, and take dietary advice from respected organizations or qualified practitioners. State registered dieticians usually operate within hospitals or in conjunction with GPs; nutritionists or nutritional therapists usually operate privately, and should hold a degree or diploma, be registered with a governing body such as the Nutritional Therapy Council and hold full indemnity and liability insurance.

You can be sure that recommendations from organizations such as the Food Standards Agency or British Nutrition Foundation have been well researched and substantiated, and provide good advice regarding a healthy, balanced diet. Recommendations are based upon foods from each of the five food groups.

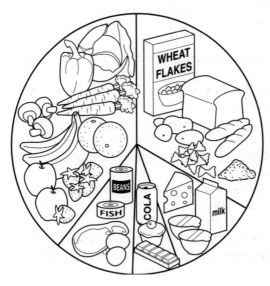

Figure 1.1 Five food groups.

(Diagram based upon the Balance of Good Health guidelines outlined by the Health Education Authority and revised by the Food Standards Agency.)

The 'food plate' in Figure 1.1 divided into five food groups:

▶ *starchy carbohydrates (bread, other cereals and potatoes)*
▶ *fruit and vegetables*
▶ *milk and dairy foods*
▶ *meat, fish and protein alternatives*
▶ *foods containing fat and sugar.*

Foods in the largest groups (fruit and vegetables and starchy carbohydrates) should be eaten most often, with protein foods consumed two to three times daily and foods high in sugar or fat consumed in much lower amounts. The proportions on the 'plate' diagram indicate the proportions that each type of food should contribute to your diet, as indicated in the UK government's tips for a healthy diet (2005):

1 *Base your meals on starchy foods.*
2 *Eat lots of fruit and vegetables.*
3 *Eat more fish.*
4 *Cut down on saturated fat and sugar.*
5 *Try to eat less salt – no more than 6 g a day.*
6 *Get active and try to be a healthy weight.*
7 *Drink plenty of water.*
8 *Don't skip breakfast.*

However, these recommendations illustrate the basic requirements of a healthy, balanced diet; further recommendations can be made to fine tune your diet and maximize your health even more.

1 BASE YOUR MEALS ON STARCHY FOODS

Unrefined carbohydrates such as wholemeal bread or brown rice contain higher levels of fibre, minerals and vitamins than their white alternatives and are therefore much more nutritious and healthy. Such foods have a low glycaemic index indicating a slower absorption rate or lower glucose content – find out more about using the glycaemic index in Chapter 7. Choosing carbohydrate foods with a slower absorption rate will provide a more sustained energy release, helping you to avoid snacking on sugary foods between meals. Basing each meal on starchy foods is easily done, and incorporating these additional tips will provide an even healthier diet.

For example:

▶ *Porridge, muesli or wholewheat toast for breakfast.*
▶ *A wholemeal sandwich or mixed bean salad for lunch.*
▶ *Brown rice risotto or potatoes in an evening meal.*

2 EAT LOTS OF FRUIT AND VEGETABLES

Although official recommendations are to eat five servings of
fruit and vegetables daily, most experts agree that this represents
the minimum we should be consuming, and many organizations
such as the National Cancer Institute are now promoting seven
servings (for women) and nine servings (for men) daily. However,
many of us fail to consume the recommended 'five a day', with
average consumption in some parts of the UK thought to be less
than one portion a day. The National Diet and Nutrition Survey
(2002) shows that although fruit and vegetable consumption
has increased over the past few years, the average is still less
than three portions a day with men eating 2.7 and women
2.9 portions.

What is a portion?
- ▶ *A cereal bowl-sized portion of salad.*
- ▶ *A medium sized apple or similar fruit.*
- ▶ *Three heaped tablespoons of berries, peas or beans.*

Insight: What else can I include in my 'five a day'?
- ▶ *Frozen, dried and tinned fruit or vegetables (although
  ideally the majority of fruits and vegetables eaten should
  be fresh)*
- ▶ *100 per cent fruit or vegetable juices or smoothies*
- ▶ *Beans and pulses also count, but only one portion of
  each of these should contribute to your five portions
  each day*

Remember that a portion size is approximately the size of your
palm, and eating a wide range of foods will provide a greater
range of nutrients, making sure that you consume all the vitamins
and minerals you need for good health. This group of foods is
also where most of the health-promoting phytonutrients (plant
nutrients) are found, proven to reduce the risk of illnesses such as
heart disease and cancer. Find out more about the phytonutrients
in Chapter 3.

Remember!

Foods such as potatoes and yams don't count towards your 'five a day' as these provide a source of starchy carbohydrates for energy rather than a rich source of vitamins, minerals and phytonutrients.

However, eating five servings of fruit or vegetables daily is still easy to achieve, and using fresh, organic produce and eating a wide variety will provide even more health benefits.

Insight: How to get your five a day
- *Include fruit with cereals and fresh fruit juice for breakfast.*
- *Add salad vegetables to sandwiches or eat salad for lunch.*
- *Include at least two vegetables in your evening meal. Simple!*

3 EAT MORE FISH

Current recommendations to include fish in the diet are as follows:

- *Consume at least two portions of fish a week, one of which is oily fish.*
- *Men and post-menopausal women should eat up to four portions of oily fish a week.*
- *A lower intake is currently advised for other women in order to limit placental exposure to toxic compounds that may be present in some fish – dioxins and polychlorinated biphenyls (PCBs).*

What are the oily fish?

Salmon, herring, mackerel, kippers, trout, sardines, pilchards, tuna, anchovies, swordfish...

Higher fish consumption is part of the so-called 'Mediterranean diet', and has been linked with reduced heart disease, lower cholesterol levels and increased cognitive (mental) function – find out more about this in Chapter 8. Although consuming tinned fish such as tuna or salmon provides some health benefits, many of the essential fatty acids are lost in the canning process, so tinned fish is a step in the right direction, but fresh, un-farmed or organic fish is the best option.

Follow these tips to include more fish in your diet.

Insight: Eat more fish for the benefits of a Mediterranean diet

▶ *Enjoy kedgeree or sardines on toast for brunch or lunch.*
▶ *Add salmon or tuna to sandwiches instead of cheese, egg or meat.*
▶ *Swap meat for fish in at least two evening meals.*

4 CUT DOWN ON SATURATED FAT AND SUGAR

Saturated fat is found predominantly in meats, full-fat dairy produce and many refined bakery products such as cakes and biscuits. This type of fat has been linked with obesity, diabetes, heart disease and some types of cancer. Although we need some fat in the diet, the type of fats we need for health are the longer chain, polyunsaturated fats found in fish, nuts and seeds, so we should try to limit our consumption of foods that are rich in saturated or processed fats such as hydrogenated and trans fatty acids. This is simple to do – try adjusting your diet as follows to reduce the 'bad' fats in your diet.

Insight: How to reduce your fat intake

▶ *Swap full-fat milk to semi-skimmed, skimmed, oat or rice milk.*
▶ *Add salmon, tuna or peppered mackerel to sandwiches and salads instead of cheese and fatty meats.*
▶ *Cut back on biscuits, cakes and pastries to reduce your fat – and calorie – intake.*

In addition to limiting the amount of fat that we eat, we should also try to curb our intake of sugar. Many people have a sweet tooth, but over quite a short period of time you can easily reduce your sugar intake. High sugar consumption is linked with obesity, dental disease and diabetes. It can play havoc with your blood sugar levels, creating more cravings for sugary snacks. Try to reduce your sugar intake with these tips, and find out more about how to control blood sugar levels in Chapter 7.

> **Insight: Watch out for hidden sugar**
> Check the labels on fizzy drinks, sweets, chocolate and foods with hidden added sugar – avoid foods containing more than 15 g of sugars per 100 g, and watch out for added ingredients ending in '-ose' as these are usually sugars, for example, maltose, dextrose or glucose.

Other ways to reduce sugar intake:

▶ *Gradually reduce the amount of sugar you add to tea or coffee until you don't need any at all.*
▶ *Try sliced banana or ripe avocado on toast instead of jam, honey or marmalade.*

5 TRY TO EAT LESS SALT – NO MORE THAN 6 g A DAY

Although it contains no calories, and is therefore often ignored by slimming clubs and weight-loss books, a high salt intake is detrimental to good health (and can also affect our weight through increased water retention). High salt (sodium chloride) consumption has been linked with hypertension, with coronary heart disease as well as some cancers, and a diet low in salt and high in fruit and vegetables has been proven to significantly reduce blood pressure. Fruit and vegetables are naturally low in sodium and rich in potassium, a mineral that helps to counteract the effects of sodium in the body. If you crave salty foods, this can be a sign that you are consuming too much sodium (salt), but as with sugar, your taste for salty foods will reduce as you decrease your salt intake. There are lots of ways to reduce salt intake – stopping adding salt to cooking and to your food is a great start! However, approximately three quarters of the salt we eat is hidden in the foods we buy, so checking food labels will help to reduce your salt consumption:

▶ *Watch out for high-salt foods that don't necessarily taste salty, such as cheese, bread and pizza.*
▶ *Eat plenty of potassium-rich foods to counteract the effects of sodium – fill up on fruit, vegetables and juices.*

Insight: Check food labels for hidden salt

Start checking the salt content on tinned and packaged foods and choose low-salt products. A high-salt food contains more than 1.5 g of salt per 100 g (or 0.6 g sodium per 100 g), and a low-salt food contains 0.3 g salt or less per 100 g (or 0.1 g sodium).

How to work out salt and sodium content

It's easier to monitor how much salt (rather than sodium) you are consuming to try to stay below 6 g a day, but some food labels may list sodium rather than salt content. You can calculate the amount of salt in a food by multiplying the sodium content by 2.5. For example, if a portion of food contains 0.8 g sodium, it will contain about 2 g of salt.

6 GET ACTIVE AND TRY TO BE A HEALTHY WEIGHT

Excess weight contributes to diabetes, heart disease and some cancers and also puts a strain on joints, adding to the risk of arthritis. Exercise not only uses up calories and raises your metabolic rate, but has also been shown to be the most effective way of maintaining a healthy body weight when done in conjunction with a healthy diet. There's no doubt that exercise plays an important part in helping us to balance the scales; Chapter 2 contains everything you need to know in order to reduce body fat levels and manage your weight, but in the meantime, try out these tips to increase your activity or start exercising:

> ▸ *Find a type of exercise that you enjoy, or you will never keep it up!*
> ▸ *Exercise with a partner, a friend or join a fitness class or club – research shows we are 22 per cent more likely to be successful at sticking with regular exercise when we exercise with others.*
> ▸ *Set yourself a monthly goal of how many exercise sessions or exercise minutes you will achieve – you're 20 per cent more likely to succeed if you have a goal!*

7 DRINK PLENTY OF WATER

Water is essential for life, yet most of us are consistently dehydrated (check out the symptoms of dehydration in Chapter 7). Water has many essential roles in the body: it enables our body to utilize the energy in foods, it regulates body temperature, helps us to eliminate waste products from the body, and is needed for digestion and muscular contraction, to name just a few. Although we get a lot of our fluid requirements from the foods that we eat (for example, from milk, soups, fruit) we should also be drinking at least a litre of water a day.

Insight: Working out how much water you really need

More accurate fluid requirements can be calculated using either body weight or calorie intake.

1 *Drink 35 ml per kg or 2.2 lbs of your body weight – for example, if you weigh 60 kg, you need about 2100 ml (2.1 litres) a day.*
2 *Drink one litre for every 1000 calories consumed.*

Chapter 6 offers tips on increasing the quantity of water you drink, but for now, consider these tips to maximize the quality of your water.

- *Jug or tap filters remove chemicals and metals such as lead and aluminium from the water supply – installing a filter to the pipe under the sink is the most effective way to ensure that all water is filtered, including that used for cooking.*
- *If you are drinking large amounts of tap water, it might be an idea to check that you haven't got old lead pipes in the kitchen which could be leaking lead into your water supply.*
- *If drinking bottled mineral water, still water, rather than sparkling, is a better option in order to avoid taking in extra carbon dioxide (this gas, which creates the bubbles in fizzy drinks, is what we breathe out and is an end product of respiration and energy metabolism – any additional carbon dioxide taken in has to be removed via the circulation, skin and lungs). Choose a mineral water with a low sodium and nitrate content, and check that it doesn't contain any added flavourings or sweeteners.*

8 DON'T SKIP BREAKFAST

Breakfast is said to be the most important meal of the day as it provides energy after a night of fasting (hence the word, breakfast!). Without breakfast we soon find our energy levels flagging and reach for caffeine or sugary snacks to keep going. Although these might do the job, they are unlikely to offer many healthy nutrients or long-term energy, and often create a poor eating pattern with caffeine- or sugar-fixes throughout the day providing energy boosts. This type of diet does not promote healthy eating, and can be the undoing of a healthy eating plan. Set yourself up for the day with these suggestions.

Breakfast options
- *Porridge is a great breakfast option as it releases energy very slowly and will give you energy right up to lunchtime.*
- *No time for breakfast? Fruit comes ready-packaged in its own skin, and is easily eaten on the go. Although not as nutritious as fresh fruit, packaged fruit salads are available in all supermarkets – how much easier can it get?*

► *Can't face breakfast? Try a fruit smoothie or a drink of juice – even though these drinks are packed with a simple sugar called fructose (fruit sugar), this provides a much slower release of energy than the glucose found in fruits so it will keep you going for longer than you anticipate. You can always top up energy levels with a cereal or nut bar later in the morning when you have more of an appetite.*

So, there are some basic guidelines for healthy eating along with tips to make your diet even healthier, but you may feel that you need more specific guidelines for particular health benefits. So now it's time to find out what you really want from your diet. Are you ready for optimum nutrition, or just looking for enhanced health benefits within a realistic time frame, budget and lifestyle?

Optimum nutrition

It has been said that there are no 'junk diets', only junk foods. In other words, you can eat one or two foods of a less nutritious nature without having an unhealthy diet. In today's lifestyle where time is at a premium, food choice almost limitless and family or social pressures constantly affecting our choice of foods, a healthy diet for most of us is all about balance and moderation. An 'optimum nutrition' diet is one that provides all the nutrients you need for continued good health. It doesn't include caffeine or alcohol, refined sugars or bakery goods, tinned and packaged foods, ready meals and take-aways or added salt or sauces.

Although many people like the idea of following an optimum nutrition diet, for most of us it's unrealistic. And you know what happens to unrealistic diets … they last as long as our will-power (which is usually between three days and three weeks!). So it's crunch time … time to be honest and decide not only what you want from your diet and how much you would like to improve your health, but also what you can realistically achieve.

Do you have the time, inclination and budget to buy and prepare organic foods? Do you want to sip on mineral water whilst friends share a bottle of wine? Maybe you would just like to make a few changes in your diet to look and feel younger? We all have different priorities, and it is your priorities that will shape your diet.

If improved health is your priority, it may be important enough for an overhaul of your current eating habits. Using the chapters in this book you may decide to kick start your new regime with a detox, follow a superfoods diet and eat organic produce. If you would love to eat more healthily but lack time, motivation or are on a budget, there are hundreds of tips throughout this book giving you quick, effective and inexpensive ways to improve your eating habits without breaking the bank.

The good news is that there are hundreds of ways to improve your diet and follow a lifetime eating plan that promises better health without having to stick to an optimum nutrition diet. Of course, the more changes you make and the healthier your diet is, the better your health and quality of life will be.

So, on a scale of 1 to 10, where 1 = junk diet and 10 = optimum nutrition, you need to decide two things:

- *Where are you now?*
- *Where do you want to be?*

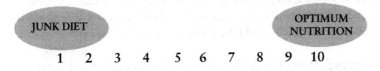

Figure 1.2 Junk diet to optimum nutrition scale.

In order to help you decide what your starting point is, have a go at this quick quiz. It will help you to identify where your diet may need the most adjustment, and your final result will give you a score on the optimum nutrition scale.

Nutrition quiz

How many servings of fruit and vegetables do you eat a day?
  a) One or less, and unlikely to be fresh fruit or vegetables
  b) Two to three
  c) Four or five
  d) I always eat five or more servings a day

How much water do you drink each day?
  a) None
  b) Only if I am thirsty, or in coffee and tea or fizzy drinks
  c) A couple of glasses daily
  d) At least eight glasses a day every day

What sort of carbohydrates do you eat?
  a) Croissants, doughnuts or teacakes
  b) French bread, white bread and white rice
  c) Granary and seed breads
  d) Wholemeal bread, brown rice and wholewheat pasta

What type of protein foods do you regularly eat?
  a) Corned beef, beef burgers or mostly processed meat or fish products
  b) Yoghurts, milk, cheese, meat products (bacon, sausages, etc.)
  c) Mainly red meats – pork, beef, lamb – with very little fish
  d) Mainly fresh fish, soya, nuts, and some organic meat

What type of fats do you consume?
  a) Lard or dripping, salad dressings and sauces, margarine and biscuits
  b) I use butter, cook with vegetable oils and eat a limited amount of bakery products containing refined fats (biscuits, pastries, etc.)
  c) I use vegetable oils for cooking and use low fat spreads
  d) Olive oil for cooking, vegetable oils for salad dressings, and avoid trans fatty acids and hydrogenated fats found in biscuits, pastries, etc.

Which of the following types of fibre do you regularly eat?
  a) White bread and breakfast cereals (corn flakes, rice krispies)
  b) Bran
  c) Wholewheat cereals such as Weetabix and wholemeal bread
  d) Fruit, vegetables, brown rice and oats

How much alcohol do you drink? (A unit is approximately a 125 ml glass of wine, a measure of spirits or half a pint of beer, depending upon the strength of the alcoholic beverage)
  a) Above 14 units (21 for men) weekly, drinking either every day or binge drinking at the weekend
  b) Between 10 to 14 units a week (15 to 21 for men)
  c) Between 5 to 10 units a week with alcohol-free days (for either sex)
  d) Under 5 units a week with alcohol free days

How many drinks of coffee, tea or caffeinated fizzy drinks do you drink each day?
  a) Over 6 cups daily
  b) 3–5 cups daily
  c) 1–2 cups daily
  d) None at all

How often do you eat sweets, crisps or other refined convenience/ready-made foods?
  a) In every meal or several times a day
  b) At least once in the day
  c) A few times through the week
  d) Rarely – only at special occasions or when there is no other option available

How many meals do you eat each day?
  a) I often miss meals and have coffee, tea or chocolate/snacks instead
  b) One or two meals – I miss breakfast and eat mostly in the evening
  c) Usually three meals including breakfast
  d) I eat regularly throughout the day including breakfast and healthy snacks

HOW DID YOU SCORE?

Mostly a):

You do need to change your diet to a healthier one. This would involve limiting the use of convenience foods, reducing salt and sugar intake, and drinking less coffee, tea and/or alcohol. Increase your servings of fresh fruit and vegetables and eat regularly throughout the day.

Place on the optimum nutrition scale – probably two to three!

Mostly b):

Some changes need to be made – look at the questions which you answered b) or a) to, and try to improve specifically on those areas. Altering different areas of your diet slowly without too many drastic changes is the best way to adopt a healthy diet and improve your health.

Place on the optimum nutrition scale – probably four to five!

Mostly c):

You eat a better diet than many people, but would still benefit from a few more changes. Most of your diet is fairly healthy, you may just need to cut back on anti-nutrients such as coffee, tea, alcohol and sugar, or address specific questions that you answered a), b) or c) to.

Place on the optimum nutrition scale – six to seven!

Mostly d):

Well done! You are already close to eating an optimum nutrition diet. Look back at the questions you answered a), b), or c) to, and now try to improve on those particular aspects of your diet.

Place on the optimum nutrition scale – seven plus!

So now you know how good (or bad) your diet is, and have identified the areas that need most attention, time for a quick reality check …

DECIDING WHERE YOU WANT TO BE

Remember, optimum nutrition isn't for everyone! If you enjoy a cup of coffee, relish a glass of wine and feel that your weekly take-away enriches your weekend (and life), then wanting to be at number ten on the scale is unrealistic. Balance and moderation in life and in our diet is important – we don't have to eat organic, raw, unprocessed foods all the time to be able to live a reasonably healthy life. Other things to consider would be the environments you live and work in, as high levels of stress and a polluted atmosphere increase our requirements for a nutrient-rich diet, as do habits such as smoking and drinking alcohol.

So, consider the following questions before you begin your journey towards (but not necessarily to) optimum nutrition.

1 *Do I have a high stress lifestyle?*
2 *How polluted is the environment in the area that I live?*
3 *How many time-saving processed foods do I eat (tinned, packet, sealed foods, ready meals, ready-made sauces, confectionary, etc.)?*
4 *What sort of dietary changes could I embrace without detrimentally affecting my family and social life?*
5 *What sort of food does my family eat? Would my changes in diet affect them?*
6 *How would my religion or moral beliefs affect my decision to eat or omit certain foods?*
7 *Do I smoke?*
8 *Do I drink alcohol?*

All of these things affect your health, the level of nutrients you need, and the level of ease with which you will adjust your eating habits.

As with all lifestyle adjustments, it's important to make changes in stages. If you decide you are currently at level three, aim to make one or two changes in your diet to get to level four. Once these changes are established as a normal habit (this will take several weeks and may take a couple of months for some changes to become habitual), you can make further adjustments to your diet to move to the next step. Many 'diets' go wrong because we try to make a change equivalent to moving from level one to level ten in one go! The more gradually you incorporate beneficial changes into your daily eating habits, the more likely it is that these changes will become a way of life.

Understanding the basics

Throughout this book many food nutrients are discussed – carbohydrates, fats, proteins (the macronutrients), vitamins and minerals (the micronutrients), fibre, phytonutrients, anti-oxidants. Although within each chapter you will find clear explanations of the nutrients discussed, a quick review of the main food nutrients and their classifications is included here to give you a basic understanding of what is in our food.

Most foods contain a mixture of different nutrients; it is rare for any food to contain just one macronutrient and most foods will contain some carbohydrate, some protein and some fat. However, we tend to classify foods based upon the main nutrient found within them. For example, although bread will contain some protein and usually a little fat, it is classified as a carbohydrate food because it contains mostly carbohydrates.

CARBOHYDRATES

Carbohydrates are our main source of energy, providing four calories per gram. They also provide most of our fibre, and often naturally occur with a range of vitamins and minerals. Foods rich in carbohydrates are listed below, although carbohydrates are also present in other foods. For example, most dairy produce contains carbohydrate in the form of the milk sugar, lactose.

Carbohydrate-rich foods
Breads, cereals, rice, pasta, beans, pulses, fruit, vegetables, sugars, jams.

Carbohydrate classifications
Carbohydrates may be classified as **simple** or **complex**.

▶ *Simple carbohydrates are primarily made up of sugars, or simple molecular structures called* **monosaccharides** *and* **disaccharides**. *The most common monosaccharide, and the one we use for energy, is called glucose.*
▶ *Complex carbohydrates are made up of larger molecules called* **polysaccharides**. *These create starches, and are a store of energy in plant foods such as potatoes, beans and pulses.*

Each food containing carbohydrates has a value known as the **Glycaemic Index (GI)** which relates to how quickly the carbohydrate is broken down (digested), enabling glucose to be absorbed into the bloodstream. Sugars, some fruits, and refined carbohydrates such as white bread generally have a quick absorption rate or high Glycaemic Index, whereas starchy foods such as porridge or beans have a low glycaemic index and a slow absorption rate. In addition to contributing to a healthy diet, the glycaemic index can be used to provide quick surges or sustained levels of energy, and can also be used to help with weight loss. Check out the chapters on weight loss or energy levels to find out how to use the Glycaemic Index to your advantage.

PROTEIN

Protein has many different uses in the body:

▶ *It is used for cellular growth and repair.*
▶ *It helps to form many important molecules in our body, including antibodies, hormones, neurotransmitters (chemical messengers in our brain) and enzymes.*

▶ *Proteins also transport many substances such as cholesterol (as high- or low-density lipoproteins) and oxygen (as haemoglobin) around the body.*

As with the carbohydrates, naturally-occurring protein foods often contain a range of vitamins and minerals. Protein foods are listed below, although protein is also found in other foods such as grains, which are generally classed as carbohydrates. Protein foods contain approximately four calories per gram, but although protein can be used to provide energy, it is not a preferred energy source.

Protein-rich foods
Dairy produce (milk, cheese, yoghurt), eggs, meat, fish, soya, beans and pulses.

Unlike carbohydrates, which are stored as glycogen in our muscles and liver, and fat, which is stored as adipose tissue, protein is not stored in the body, although it forms our lean tissue that can be broken down if amino acids are required to form protein molecules. An adequate protein intake is vital in the diet for continued good health.

Protein classification
Proteins are made up of molecules called amino acids, and of the 20 or so that we regularly use, eight of these are essential in the diet as we cannot manufacture them in the body.

▶ *Foods containing all eight essential amino acids are called complete protein.*
▶ *Foods lacking in one or more of the essential amino acids are known as incomplete protein.*

Complete protein foods	Incomplete protein foods
Eggs	Beans and pulses
Meat	Vegetables
Fish	Cereals and grains
Dairy foods	

Protein from soya products is the most complete vegetable protein source.

However, vegetable proteins can be combined to provide complete protein in a meal. Simply combining a grain with any type of bean will provide complete protein, as each type of food has different levels of amino acids which complement each other. This is a healthy way to consume complete protein, as vegetable protein sources do not contain the high levels of saturated fat often found in animal proteins such as meat, eggs or dairy foods.

Top tip for vegetarians and vegans
Combine grains such as wheat, corn or rice with beans or pulses for a meal containing complete protein – try chilli with beans and rice, or beans on toast.

FATS

Contrary to popular belief, not all fats are bad for you! Fats provide more than double the amount of energy (nine calories per gram) than the proteins and carbohydrates, and as such are a useful energy source, but they also have other functions:

▶ *Fats are used for insulation to keep us warm.*
▶ *They protect our internal organs.*
▶ *Fats contribute to the formation and function of our cell membranes.*
▶ *They are required to form essential compounds called prostaglandins which help to control blood pressure, immune function and inflammation.*

Two types of fatty acid are essential for many of these functions, and are therefore required in our diet – these are the omega 3 and omega 6 fatty acids. Alpha linolenic acid is the most common type of omega 3 fatty acid, and linoleic acid is the most common type of omega 6 fatty acid, so these are known as the essential fatty acids. All other types of fatty acid can be manufactured in the body from these fats, so although other types of fat can be beneficial, they are not essential. However, if any fatty acid conversion cannot be made, other types of fat may become essential for continued good health. For example, the long chain fatty acids found in fish, although not classed as essential, provide a range of health benefits, and should ideally be included in a healthy non-vegetarian diet.

Foods containing fats
Fats and oils such as butter, margarine, vegetable oils, dripping, suet and lard, and meat, fish, eggs, dairy produce, nuts, seeds, avocado, dips or sauces such as mayonnaise, salad cream or hummus.

Foods containing the essential fatty acids
▶ *Linoleic acid is found in vegetable oils, margarines, nuts and seeds.*
▶ *Linolenic acid is found in similar foods, but is only present in high amounts in fatty fish and some types of seed such as linseeds.*

Fats occur naturally with the fat soluble vitamins (A, D, E and K) and are an important dietary source of these vitamins. For example, dairy foods contain vitamin A; vitamin E is found in vegetable oils; and vitamin D in oily fish. Vitamin K, however, is found mostly in green leafy vegetables.

Foods rich in fats are listed below.

Classification of fats
Saturated fat

▶ *This is found mostly in meats, egg yolks and dairy produce.*
▶ *This type of fat is usually solid at room temperature.*
▶ *A high intake of saturated fat is linked to heart disease and obesity.*

Monounsaturated fat

▶ *This is found mostly in plant foods and oils such as avocados, nuts, seeds and olive oil.*

▶ *Monounsaturated fats are the healthiest type of oil to cook with, and olive oil has been shown to have beneficial cardiovascular properties, especially as part of a healthy, Mediterranean-type diet also high in fruit, vegetables and fish.*

Polyunsaturated fat

▶ *This is found in vegetable oils, margarines and fish.*
▶ *It is this group of fats which contains both the essential fatty acids (linolenic and linoleic) and the long chain fish oils known to be beneficial to health.*
▶ *It is best to obtain these oils directly from their natural food source by including fish, nuts, seeds and cold vegetable oils, which can be used as a salad dressing, in your diet.*
▶ *Polyunsaturated vegetable oils such as sunflower or safflower oil are not as healthy when heated, as oxygen can easily combine with them and cause free radical damage in the body. Chapter 6 discusses free radical damage in more detail.*

FIBRE

Fibre is found in most carbohydrate foods, and it travels the length of our digestive tract largely undigested, so it provides no calories. However, it does have a role to play in our diet:

▶ *Fibre helps to make us feel full, so it can contribute to a healthy weight-loss or weight-maintenance diet.*
▶ *Insoluble fibre helps to move food and the products of digestion along the digestive tract, which reduces constipation and improves bowel health.*
▶ *Soluble fibre absorbs excess cholesterol and toxins in the digestive tract, carrying them out of the body with other waste products (see Chapter 4 for more details).*

There are two types of fibre, soluble and insoluble, and we need a combination of both types for good health. Soluble fibre is found in fruits, vegetables and oats, whereas insoluble fibre is found in many grains such as rice or wheat.

Fibre-rich foods
Wholegrain breakfast cereals, brown rice, oats, fruit, vegetables, beans, pulses, nuts and seeds.

Proof that a healthy diet works

There is much research that supports the association between a healthy diet and improved health, and the dietary recommendations made throughout this book are based upon such evidence. In particular, many clinical trials as well as epidemiological studies suggest a positive association between fruit and vegetable consumption and decreased risk of heart disease and various cancers. We all know that eating fruit and vegetables is good for us, but scientific evidence really illustrates what a difference to our health a few simple dietary adjustments can make.

> **Insight**
> You can reduce your risk of coronary heart disease by 4 per cent for each additional portion per day of vegetables, and by 7 per cent for each piece of fruit eaten! Green leafy vegetables are especially good!

One of the ways that fruit and vegetables can help to reduce the risk of heart disease is by lowering blood pressure. A 'normal' blood pressure reading is 120/80 mmHg, where the first figure represents the systolic blood pressure and the second figure is the diastolic pressure (this figure tends to increase from our mid-20s as we age). One study illustrates that eating fruit and vegetables can reduce systolic and diastolic blood pressure by 8.3 and 4.1 mmHg respectively. Another great way to reduce your blood pressure is by reducing your salt intake.

Regular consumption of fruit and vegetables will also help to reduce your risk of heart disease through lowering cholesterol levels. Positive cholesterol-lowering results are repeatedly associated with apple, carrots, garlic and other foods such as

Jerusalem artichoke, chicory or asparagus – these vegetables contain a type of fibre called inulin, which is the active ingredient responsible for the cholesterol-lowering benefits.

The Mediterranean-style diet has been repeatedly linked with a decreased risk of cardiovascular disease due to reduced cholesterol and blood pressure measurements, improved glucose metabolism, and reduced damage and inflammation in artery cell walls. Each separate element of the Mediterranean-style diet contributes to better health, so combining all of these in your diet can give you a significant boost to health:

- *Increase your fish consumption.*
- *Eat more fruit and vegetables.*
- *Include nuts in your diet (walnuts, almonds, Brazils, etc.).*
- *Use olive oil for cooking, dipping bread and salad dressing.*

There is no doubt that our diet affects our health and whilst individual foods or nutrients may affect specific functions in the body, some foods have multiple health-promoting benefits (the superfoods), and a combination of several healthy eating habits will have a cumulative effect upon your health and well-being.

Each chapter in this book covers a different aspect of healthy eating, and each features its own food heroes – cruciferous vegetables to aid detoxification, garlic as a renowned superfood, anti-oxidants to combat ageing, or oily fish to support mental function. However, you will also discover that many foods benefit us in several different ways, and building your diet around these foods will bring multiple benefits, whatever your goal is. You will also be pleasantly surprised at how easy it can be to improve your diet, with a little bit of know-how, helpful practical tips, and quick and easy recipes.

THINGS TO REMEMBER

So, remember the basics:

- *Base your meals on starchy foods.*

- *Eat lots of fruit and vegetables.*

- *Eat more fish.*

- *Cut down on saturated fat.*

- *Cut down on sugar.*

- *Eat less salt.*

- *Try to maintain a healthy weight.*

- *Drink plenty of water.*

- *Don't skip breakfast.*

- *Eat a balanced and varied diet.*

2

....

Eat to lose weight

In this chapter you will learn:
- *how to set an achievable weight loss goal*
- *how to reduce your calorie intake and increase energy expenditure*
- *how to maintain weight loss for life.*

The biggest question on everyone's lips is how to lose weight and keep it off! The solution is simple, but not necessarily easy! However, with a little know-how and helpful tips, you can create your own weight-loss plan and go on to balance calorie intake and expenditure for lifelong weight maintenance.

Reasons for weight gain

There are three key reasons why we gain weight:

1 *We eat too many high-calorie foods or foods with hidden calories.*
2 *Our portion sizes are too large – we may be eating the right foods but are simply eating too much of them.*
3 *We aren't active enough to use up the calories we have consumed. This is common when a change in job or lifestyle has resulted in lower activity levels and calorie intake is not adjusted accordingly.*

1   *Swapping milk to skimmed or soya milk.*
2   *Going for a 30-minute walk every day.*
3   *Reducing meat, cheese and starchy carbohydrate portion sizes and filling up on vegetables.*

The Energy Balance Equation

Weight control is simply based on something called the Energy Balance Equation as shown below.

> If energy in = energy out, weight maintenance is achieved.

So it follows that if we take in more calories than we use up, we gain weight, and if our calorie intake is lower than our expenditure, we lose weight. If your weight has been approximately the same for a while, this means you have achieved calorie balance; you are consuming the same number of calories as you are using up. Weight gain indicates that you have been taking in more calories than you need, or are not using up as many calories as you need to.

Think of it as a credit–debit arrangement. Whenever you consume extra calories, you need to add activity or exercise over and above your usual level to work off the extra food eaten! Here's a simple way of looking at weight control and the choices you have.

Weight-control choices

Choice	Result
Eat high calorie foods and tempting snacks, but don't do any extra activity.	You will put weight on as you have taken in more calories

Do additional activity or exercise to use up the extra calories in your biscuits, chips, crisps, etc.	Your weight may remain largely unchanged as you have balanced your calorie intake with energy expenditure.
Avoid high calorie foods but do no extra exercise.	You will gradually reduce your weight as you reduce calorie intake.
Avoid high calorie foods and large portions of food, AND do the extra exercise.	You will lose weight more quickly as you take in fewer calories, and create an extra deficit by using more calories during exercise.

By balancing calorie control in your favour, you will soon begin to notice a difference. This won't be an overnight result, but it should be permanent as long as you continue to maintain energy balance. You can still go out for dinner or enjoy an occasional indulgence, but by stopping habitual snacks and poor eating habits, you create the opportunity to have your cake and eat it, without unfortunate after effects!

For quicker results, limit your energy intake by following a healthy, balanced diet, and use up additional calories by maximizing the amount of activity you do every day. As you lose weight and begin to feel healthier, you'll find the extra energy and motivation to fit regular exercise into your lifestyle ... and then the results can be really uplifting!

Although achieving energy balance or creating a calorie deficit may sound simple, in order to achieve this we need to know the following information:

▶ *how many calories we need each day*
▶ *which foods or drinks are high in calories*
▶ *how the activity we do each day affects our calorie balance.*

One way to find out if you need to lose weight is to calculate your **Body Mass Index (BMI)**. However, it is important to remember that this measurement is based upon your height and weight alone, and does not take into account the amount of muscle, or lean tissue, you have. For example, if you weight train regularly, the extra muscle will increase your weight, yet you may carry less body fat than someone of the same weight as you. If your BMI seems unduly high, it may be worth having your body fat levels checked with a health and fitness professional, or using a set of scales which measure body fat as well as weight.

Calculating your Body Mass Index

1 CONVERT YOUR WEIGHT INTO KILOGRAMS

(If your scales show your weight in kilograms, then you can skip to number 2 – calculating your height in metres!).

First of all, write down your weight in pounds. For example, if you weigh 10 stones 8 lbs, multiply 10 by 14 (because there are 14 pounds in each stone), and then add on the 8 lbs to give your total weight in pounds. In this example it would be as follows:

$$10 \times 14 = 140 + 8 = 148 \text{ lbs}$$

Now convert this into kilograms by dividing it by 2.2.

For example: 148 divided by 2.2 = 67.27 kg

2 CONVERT YOUR HEIGHT INTO METRES

You can either use a conversion chart for this, or convert feet and inches into metres as follows. If you know your height in metres, you can skip to the next part where we calculate your height^2 (squared).

Write down your height in inches. For example, if you are 5 feet 5 inches tall, multiply 5 by 12 (because there are 12 inches in each foot), and then add on the extra 5 inches to give your total height in inches. In this example it would be as follows:

$5 \times 12 = 60 + 5 = 65$ inches

Now convert this into centimetres by multiplying it by 2.54.

For example: 65 multiplied by 2.54 = 165.1 cm

And now divide this by 100 to convert it into metres ...

165.1 cm divided by 100 = 1.65 metres.

Before you can calculate your Body Mass Index, you need to do a further calculation by multiplying your height in metres by the same figure again. This gives you your height^2 (squared).

Using our example of a height of 1.65 metres ...

$1.65 \times 1.65 = 2.72$ m^2.

Now you have your weight in kilograms and your height in metres^2, you can calculate your Body Mass Index.

3 BODY MASS INDEX (BMI) = WEIGHT (KG) DIVIDED BY HEIGHT (M^2)

Now divide your weight (in kg) by your height (in m^2) to give you your BMI. In this example, the Body Mass Index is calculated as follows:

67.27 kg divided by 2.72 m = 24.73.

Now check out your Body Mass Index (BMI) below.

BMI of 20–24.9 is desirable

BMI of 25–30 is considered overweight

BMI of 30+ is considered obese

BMI of 40+ is considered morbidly obese

You can also plot your weight and height on the chart below to see which category you fall into. Weight is shown at the bottom in stones/pounds, and at the top in kilograms. Remember, if you have lots of lean tissue (muscle), you may appear to be overweight when in fact you are not.

So now you have an idea of how you measure up, but before you start counting calories, let's find out how many calories you need every day.

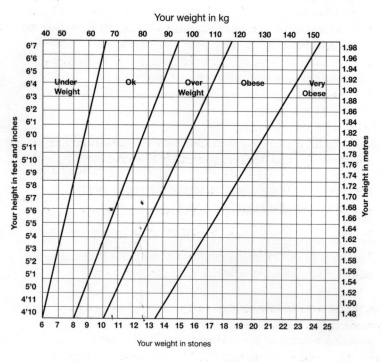

Figure 2.1 Body mass index chart.

Basal Metabolic Rate

Your Basal Metabolic Rate (BMR) is the number of calories you need each day at rest. If you are quite active you will require more calories; you can take this into account after you have worked out the basic number of calories you need each day. Although it is too time consuming for most of us to weigh the food that we eat and count calories every meal, it's worth knowing how many calories your body needs each day, as it's a common error to reduce calorie intake too low. Remember though, this is just a guideline, as the number of calories you need is also affected by your height, the amount of lean tissue (muscle) you have, and your activity levels.

CALCULATING YOUR BASAL METABOLIC RATE

1 First of all, find your age range in the tables (Male or Female) below.
2 Now multiply your weight in kilograms (kg) by the figure shown for your age.
3 Finally, add on the number at the end.

Basal Metabolic Rates (Females)

Age	Basal Metabolic Rate
10–17	Weight in kg multiplied by 13.4 + 692
18–29	Weight in kg multiplied by 14.8 + 487
30–59	Weight in kg multiplied by 8.3 + 846
60–74	Weight in kg multiplied by 9.2 + 687
75+	Weight in kg multiplied by 9.8 + 624

So, if you were female aged 40 and your weight was 67 kg, you would do the following calculation.

$67 \times 8.3 = 556.1$ and then add 846 to give a total of 1402.1 calories.

Basal Metabolic Rates (Males)

Age	Basal Metabolic Rate
10–17	Weight in kg multiplied by 17.7 + 657
18–29	Weight in kg multiplied by 15.1 + 692
30–59	Weight in kg multiplied by 11.5 + 873
60–74	Weight in kg multiplied by 11.9 + 700
75+	Weight in kg multiplied by 8.4 + 821

EXTRA CALORIES FOR ACTIVITY AND EXERCISE

You can multiply your daily calorie requirement (BMR) by 1.4 to take account of general activity during work and relaxation. Most of us would not need to adjust our calorie requirement by any more than this, although those doing regular high intensity exercise such as running four or five times weekly might multiply their BMR figure by up to 1.6 or even 1.8.

So now take your BMR calculated from the previous table, and multiply it by 1.4 to account for additional activity. Using the earlier example, we would multiply 1402 calories by 1.4 = 1963 calories needed daily.

Now you have an idea of how many calories you need each day. However, remember that this is the number of calories you need at your current weight for weight maintenance. If you want to lose weight, you will need to consume fewer calories than this.

How much weight should you lose?

Insight

A reasonable guideline for your first weight-loss goal is 5 per cent of your body weight, unless you have a BMI which places you as very obese, in which case you may be able to safely lose 10 per cent of your body weight.

CALCULATING HOW MUCH WEIGHT TO LOSE

To calculate 5 per cent of your body weight, multiply your weight in pounds (or kilograms if you prefer) by 5, then divide by 100. Using the earlier example of a body weight of 148 lbs, this gives us:

148 × 5 = 740, divided by 100 = 7.4 lbs

In this example, 7.4 lbs is 5 per cent of the person's total body weight, and is the first weight-loss goal. If you planned to lose this weight over a six-week period, you would need to lose 1.2 lbs weekly (just divide the weight-loss goal you have by 6 as follows):

7.4 lbs divided by 6 weeks = 1.2 lbs weight loss weekly.

Six to eight weeks is a good time period to use when setting short-term goals. Remember, this is just your first 'mini' weight-loss goal, and does not necessarily represent the total amount of weight you might want to lose.

If 5 per cent of your current weight divided over six weeks comes to more than a 1 lb weekly weight loss, it's worth planning the weight loss over eight weeks, or simply limiting your weekly weight loss to 1 lb, to make sure it's realistic. This is because many weight-loss goals fail if they are based upon an unachievable weekly weight loss. Any weight-lost in addition to the original goal set is a bonus! So here are some helpful guidelines to help you set your first weight-loss goal.

SETTING SUCCESSFUL WEIGHT-LOSS GOALS

The way to successful weight loss and weight maintenance is through making small changes and taking small steps. This way, your lifestyle is less disrupted and you can continue successfully. Once the new changes become a habit, you can make further changes. It is a common mistake to aim for the total weight loss you want (for example, two stones) without breaking it down into smaller goals.

Deciding on your initial weight-loss goal

This should be a weight that you can realistically lose over a six-week period. A common goal is to lose a pound or two a week. However, when you consider how much of a calorie loss you would have to achieve in order to lose two pounds a week, you may reconsider!

> **Insight**
>
> There are approximately 3,500 calories in 1 lb of fat. So to lose 2 lb of fat a week, you have to create a calorie deficit of approximately 7,000 calories over the week, or eat 1,000 calories less a day! This is a tall order for most people, and is unrealistic unless you have a lot of weight to lose, or are currently consuming a very high-calorie diet. Even losing 1 lb weekly requires a calorie deficit of 3,500 calories a week, or 500 calories daily.

Later on we'll look at your food diary to see where you might find 500 calories to cut out, but for now, let's agree on your weight-loss goal.

It's also worth considering that the less weight you have to lose, the less body fat you are likely to lose each week. So if you have a stone or less to lose, aim for a smaller loss of no more than half a pound weekly. It's better to achieve the goal you originally set, rather than begin with an unrealistic target and then fail. A loss of half a pound weekly would still create an overall weight loss of nearly half a stone over 12 weeks.

SMART GOALS

Setting SMART goals for weight loss will increase your chances of success. SMART stands for goals that are:

> *Specific*
> *Measurable*
> *Achievable*
> *Realistic*
> *Time-bound*

SETTING YOUR SMART WEIGHT-LOSS GOAL

Choose your SPECIFIC goal
This is the weight you want to be at the end of six weeks.

Make sure it's MEASURABLE
Use the same set of scales to measure your success. If you haven't got access to any weighing scales, you could choose a different goal such as a waist or hip measurement, or choose an item of clothing that you want to fit into.

Make sure your goal is ACHIEVABLE and REALISTIC
Although you will naturally want weight-loss results as quickly as possible, setting yourself a tough goal is likely to end in failure, which is de-motivating and often contributes to further weight gain. Consider this example ...

If you set a weight-loss goal to lose one stone over six weeks and lost 12 lbs you may feel disappointed because you didn't hit your weight-loss target. However, if you set a weight-loss goal of 10 lbs over six weeks and lost 12 lbs, you will feel motivated as you over-achieved your target. The weight loss is the same in both examples, but the level of motivation and feeling of achievement is different, and may affect whether you continue with your weight-loss efforts or not. The idea is not to set a goal that is easy to achieve, but to decide upon an achievable, realistic weight-loss goal.

As a general guideline, if your Body Mass Index placed you in the 'very obese' category, you may be able to lose 1–2 lbs weekly. If you were in the overweight bracket, or have approximately a stone to lose, don't aim to lose any more than 1 lb weekly.

Make it TIME-BOUND to make it work!
Decide on a date by which you will achieve your first weight-loss goal. Write it in your diary, mark it on the calendar, maybe even plan to treat yourself (not with chocolates!) when you reach your

first goal weight. Six weeks is thought to be the best period of time for successful goal setting – it's not too far away that you delay your weight-loss diet, and it is close enough to keep you motivated. However, if you have an important event that you would like to lose weight for, such as a wedding, holiday or social occasion, you might want to use this date as your goal if it's within two months.

So now you have your goal, you know what weight you want to be in a specific number of weeks' time and you know how you will measure your success. Now let's take a look at how you're going to do it!

You have three options:

1 *reducing your calorie intake*
2 *using up more calories through activity and exercise*
3 *eating less and exercising more.*

---

1 Reducing your calorie intake

Rather than begin randomly cutting foods out of your diet (like many fad diets), for long-term success, take a more considered approach. If you cut out all the foods you enjoy eating, your weight loss will be short lived. Experts say that the typical 'fad' diet lasts between three days and three weeks – the same length of time as our differing will-power!

The first thing to think about is whether you eat a lot of high calorie foods. You may have a good idea of which foods are high in calories – fatty meats, spreads and oils, alcohol, cakes, biscuits and confectionary, for example, but knowing which foods to avoid and actually doing it are two different things! One of the best ways to help you cut calories from your diet is by keeping a food diary. This enables you to write down everything that you eat and drink, figure out where the excess calories are, and then choose how to reduce your daily intake.

KEEPING A FOOD DIARY

A typical food diary is shown below: you can either copy this or make up one of your own. You can begin completing a food diary from today, or write in the meals you know you have eaten over the last few days. Be careful trying to memorize what you have consumed; research shows that we often forget snacks and drinks. However, your food diary isn't going to be used to calculate daily calorie intake, but simply to help you identify foods or habits which are contributing to your weight gain.

Food diary

Meal	Mon	Tues	Wed	Thurs	Fri	Sat	Sun
Breakfast							
Lunch							
Evening							
Supper							
Snacks							
Fluids							

Now it's time to figure out where the hidden calories are in your weekly diet, and which foods you want to reduce to give you the weight loss you want.

Some foods, such as butter, cream or fatty meat, are known to be high in calories, but others may come as a surprise. Check out the table on the next page to see the approximate calorie count of some foods.

If a food is high in calories, it doesn't mean you have to avoid it completely, but if it is one of your weekly (or even daily) staples, it could be having a significant effect on your waistline. Simply cutting out a couple of glasses of wine in the evening could provide half the calorie deficit you need to lose 1 lb of weight a week. If you made no other changes, you could lose approximately half a pound a week just from this one change.

Calories in certain foods

Food	Average calories in a portion
Peanut butter	Spreading peanut butter on a couple of slices of bread or crackers will add an extra 300 calories to a snack attack!
A packet of sandwiches	Most pre-packed sandwiches pack a heavy punch of around 600 calories, providing about a quarter of the energy most of us need in a day – before you add a packet of crisps and a drink!
Hummus	Dipping your raw vegetables into a dip like hummus can undo your efforts at choosing a lower calorie snack – a typical serving can provide well over 300 calories.
Cheese	You may already know that cheese is high in fat and calories, but did you realize that just a sandwich can contain over 400 calories?
Potato skins starter with a garlic mayo dip	This tasty starter contains 353 calories – before you even tuck into your main meal!
Prawn crackers	Munching away on the free bag of prawn crackers your local take-away has given you can have you consuming an extra 400 calories on top of your take-away!

Double cream	Okay, we all know this is one to avoid on any diet, but it's really worth swapping for Greek yoghurt or fromage frais when you know a helping packs in a whopping 372 calories.
Alcohol	A couple of glasses of wine each evening could be adding 250 calories daily ... or 1,750 calories over the week!

You may look at your diet and think you can easily reduce your intake by 500 calories a day or you may already be following a reduced-calorie diet or eating healthily, and think there is really no room to reduce your intake any lower. You certainly shouldn't consider reducing your calorie intake below the BMR figure you calculated earlier.

Here are some tips to help you choose how to adapt your diet.

Reducing your calorie intake by 250 calories a day can give you a weekly weight loss of half a pound. Do this by ...

▶ *cutting out two large glasses of wine each evening*
▶ *not adding yoghurt to cereals or smoothies*
▶ *cutting out a packet of crisps each day*
▶ *cutting out two biscuits with tea/coffee twice daily.*

Reducing your calorie intake by 500 calories a day can give you a weight loss of 1 lb weekly. Do this by ...

▶ *cutting out a bottle of wine each evening*
▶ *cutting out four slices of bread with butter or margarine*
▶ *cutting out the equivalent of three to four matchbox size chunks of cheddar or a similar amount of full-fat cream cheese*
▶ *not having a weekly take-away!*

Of course, the easiest way to do this is by adjusting lots of things in your diet, so that you don't miss any one thing too much.

By reducing alcohol intake, swapping full-fat dairy foods like yoghurt and cheese for low-fat products, not eating buttered bread with meals, and cutting down on confectionary and take-away meals, you can significantly reduce your calorie intake and simultaneously eat a healthier diet.

Have a look at the examples below:

Calorie-saving chart

Food	Calories	Alternative	Calories	CALORIE SAVING
Double cream serving	372	Greek yoghurt	69	303
Whole milk with cereals	66	Skimmed milk	32	34
Jacket potato	272	Sweet potato	170	102

So, even these three simple changes could give you the following calorie saving …

Swapping a normal potato for a sweet potato twice weekly …

2 × 102 = 204 calorie saving

Swapping whole milk to skimmed milk on cereals seven days a week …

7 × 34 = 238 calorie saving

Swapping a helping of double cream at the weekend to Greek yoghurt …

1 × 303 = 303 calorie saving.

Total weekly calorie saving = 745 calories!

These changes alone could create a weight loss of 1 lb over four and a half weeks. That might not seem much, but making changes like this to your diet has three benefits:

1 *These changes also promote good health.*
2 *You won't feel like you are on a diet making small changes like this.*
3 *In conjunction with other similar dietary adjustments, you can easily and steadily lose weight.*

Real-life success

Maddie chose to change individual aspects of her diet one at a time. Once each change had become habitual, she moved onto the next one, gradually losing weight as she made changes. Once she had changed everything apart from sacrificing her evening glass of wine, she chose to keep this indulgence as she had lost two stones in weight and was happy with her new figure.

There are lots of ways to reduce your calorie intake. Have a look at the sections below and choose tips that you think might help you. When new eating habits become habitual, look at the list again and choose some more.

TIPS TO HELP YOU REDUCE CALORIE INTAKE

▶ *Eat off smaller plates – this helps you reduce portion size, and you'll still feel as if you have had a plate full of food.*
▶ *Throw leftovers away immediately so that you don't start eating them later.*
▶ *Drink plenty of water throughout the day so that you don't mistake thirst for hunger pangs!*

- *By eating regularly you will stabilize blood sugar levels, helping you to avoid cravings and over-eating. Eat more often, but reduce the amount that you eat at meal times, and snack on low-calorie fruit or raw vegetables.*
- *Leave the last couple of mouthfuls on your plate, or hold back on that last serving!*
- *Eat slowly! This gives your body a chance to tell you that you are full and should stop eating! Many of us have already finished our meal before this 'message' is sent!*
- *Listen to your body! When you begin to feel full, stop eating!*
- *Sip water between mouthfuls to slow down your eating.*
- *Doing something else whilst we eat – like watching TV – takes attention away from our meal, making us more likely to eat quickly and not notice how much we have consumed. Sit down at the table and enjoy your food.*
- *Keep tempting foods out of sight! Each time you see the biscuits or chocolate, you will be tempted to eat them. Store foods like this in cupboards that you don't often use. Out of sight, out of mind!*
- *Eat light at night! The later you eat in the evening and the bigger the meal, the less likely you are to use up the calories you've eaten.*
- *Get the family involved. If others in the household are eating a healthier diet with you, it becomes easier for you to stick to it.*
- *Fill up on fibre. It contains no digestible calories, and a high-fibre meal will fill you up, making you want to eat less! Try the following to increase fibre intake … change white rice to brown, swap refined breakfast cereals for porridge and add beans and pulses to stews and casseroles.*

Eating out needn't undo all that hard work!

- *Don't feel left out when friends are ordering dessert – order a coffee instead so you have something in front of you to enjoy while they're piling on the calories!*
- *Share a pud! Many people feel the need to finish a meal with something sweet – halve the dessert and halve the calories. You'll be doing your pudding partner a favour too!*

- *Don't starve yourself all day if you're going out for dinner. Research shows that we are more likely to overeat and choose high-fat, high-sugar and high-calorie foods when we're hungry, making it easy to consume more than any calories you've saved through the day.*

It all starts when you go shopping …

- *Don't go shopping if you are hungry. With a low blood sugar level, you will fill your trolley with sugary, refined carbohydrate foods that you wouldn't usually choose and you know once you've bought them, you'll eat them!*
- *Make a supermarket shopping list and stick to it!*
- *Go shopping with a friend or partner who has your best interests at heart – they can step in when your willpower slips.*
- *If temptation is too much, get someone else to shop for you, or shop online where you can't see the biscuits or smell the fresh bread.*

Be prepared

- *Plan your meals in advance for the week so you know what you will be eating and nothing is left to chance.*
- *Take a walk at lunchtime – and pick up a healthy lunch. The extra exercise will help those weight-loss goals and the walk will get you away from the work canteen!*
- *Take control of what you eat! Prepare your lunch for the next day by making extra rice or pasta, or baking an extra potato for your evening meal and adding salad and tinned fish for a nutritious, low-calorie lunch.*

Drink less alcohol – it contains almost as many calories as fat!

- *Spritzers last longer than just wine and water down your calorie consumption!*
- *Alternate alcoholic drinks with mineral water or juice to halve the calories.*
- *Arrive fashionably late and miss the first round!*

- *Don't go out thirsty – the first couple of drinks won't touch the sides! Drink lots of water throughout the day to avoid trying to quench a thirst with the first drinks of the evening.*
- *Offer to drive!*
- *Decide to stay within a certain number of alcohol units each week. Work out how many alcohol units you usually drink, then reduce it. Remember, a unit is a small glass of wine, half a pint or a measure of spirits. It is recommended that women don't exceed 14 units a week and men stay below 21 units.*
- *Have alcohol-free days.*

PORTION SIZES

In a civilization where food shortages are virtually unknown, most of us overeat, seduced by the smell, sight and taste of food. Many research projects have shown that we naturally eat less food in the following circumstances:

- *when we are eating fewer different foods in one meal*
- *if we slow down the speed of our eating and listen to our body*
- *if less food is available, for example, if we eat off smaller plates.*

Insight

Watch out! We tend to eat more if:

- *we eat quickly*
- *we use larger plates or dishes*
- *we have missed a meal, or reduced our calorie intake by too much*
- *we are eating lots of different foods, for example at a buffet*
- *we are distracted by something other than our meal, for example, the television.*

What happens to the extra food?
Our body can only metabolize so much food in one go, whether we eat carbohydrates (rice, pasta, vegetables), protein foods (meat, fish), or fats (cream, butter, oils). Some fats have roles in the body, but much of the saturated fat we eat has just two fates …

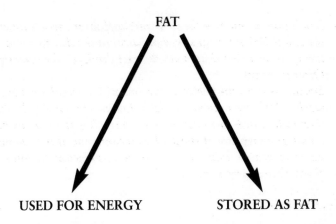

FAT

USED FOR ENERGY   **STORED AS FAT**

Carbohydrates and proteins have many useful roles in the body, but excess that cannot be used (or stored, in the case of carbohydrates) may be converted to fat and stored as adipose tissue. So you could be eating a fat-free diet, and still lay down excess body fat if you ate too much carbohydrate or protein. Alcohol follows the same fate: once metabolized in the liver, if it isn't used up for energy, it is converted into fat and may be stored as adipose tissue!

What difference does portion size make?

The answer is 'all the difference'! You may be eating a healthy, balanced diet, but simply eating too much during each meal. Once you get used to eating a certain amount, for example, pouring a certain amount of cereal into a bowl every morning, it can be difficult to break that habit.

Common mistakes
Large servings of cereals, pasta and rice are common. Although these are generally healthy foods, consuming too much in one meal increases the likelihood of the excess carbohydrate being converted

into fat and stored. A large cereal bowl can hold a 200 g portion of cereal, providing an average 579 calories (without any milk, sugar, yoghurt or fruit added). Alternatively, 50 g, which is a reasonable portion size, provides 145 calories. Making this change means you are consuming 434 CALORIES FEWER EVERY DAY – almost enough to create a weight loss of 1 lb weekly!

However, breakfast should be sustaining enough to provide energy through to lunchtime to prevent snacking on sugary foods, so reduce your portion sizes slowly, and snack on fruit, raw vegetables or rice cakes mid-morning if you get hungry.

So it's easy to see where those extra calories may be coming from – portion sizes a little too large, hidden high-calorie foods and too much variety in every meal!

Insight

Check out your dinner portions for a quick win – a large (350 g) serving of pasta could weigh in at 557 calories (without the sauce, etc.) but a 150 g serving provides 239 calories, and a saving of 318 extra calories. This change alone could result in a weekly weight loss of over half a pound!

2 Using up more calories through activity and exercise

Now let's explore how you can lose weight by using up more calories through activity and exercise. This section is for you if …

▶ *you found it difficult to find ways to reduce your current calorie consumption*
▶ *you would prefer to keep some 'treats' in your weekly diet and use activity and exercise to create a calorie deficit.*

There are many ways of using up more calories throughout the week. Regular exercise is the best way to use up energy, but increasing your activity throughout the day can also help. Even if you managed to exercise for an hour daily, there are still another 23 hours in each day (15 if you deduct eight hours for sleeping!) during which you can help yourself to lose weight. Here are some ways in which you could fit extra activity into your daily routine. As with the tips to reduce calories, choose the options which will suit you the most, as you'll be more likely to stick with them.

WAYS TO BE MORE ACTIVE

▶ *Use the stairs rather than the lift – especially if you work or live somewhere with stairs and can make this a regular calorie burner!*
▶ *Don't send emails to office colleagues! Bring back the art of conversation – walk to their desk to give them a message!*
▶ *Don't drive around car parks until a space right next to the door is free! Park further away and walk! Even better, leave the car at home!*
▶ *Get off the bus a stop early.*
▶ *Walk the children to school.*
▶ *Walk to the shops instead of sending someone else!*
▶ *Take up an active hobby such as dancing or gardening.*
▶ *Take the dog (or other people's dogs!) for a walk.*
▶ *Don't put the housework off! It may be boring but vacuuming, dusting and even ironing can all notch up reasonable calorie expenditure.*
▶ *Keep an activity log with your food diary. Jot down every extra activity you do each day. This will motivate you to try to do something extra every day, just so you can write it down!*

However, nothing can beat the benefits of regular exercise for helping to reduce body weight. Although many people begin exercising to lose weight, if you choose an exercise that you enjoy, you'll feel healthier and fitter, and also enjoy the social benefits that many types of exercise bring. Weight loss often just becomes an added bonus!

If you plan to lose 1 lb a week, you need to create a calorie deficit of 500 calories a day. But how long would you need to exercise to do this? It depends on how much effort you put in, and which type of exercise you choose to do. The more effort you put in, the more calories you use up, so you can exercise for a shorter period of time. For example, you would need to walk at a fast pace for almost two hours to use up approximately 500 calories, but you could use up the same amount of calories in a 45 minute run.

Of course, the number of calories you use up is individual; your weight, body composition and fitness level all affect how much energy you use up. But as a guideline, here are some other examples of workouts that would use up approximately 500 calories:

- *45 minutes on a step machine in the gym.*
- *Just over an hour playing a reasonably hard game of tennis.*
- *Over two hours of golf (without the buggy!).*
- *One hour of cycling.*

Of course the main thing about exercise is to make it a regular occurrence!

TIPS TO HELP YOU USE UP MORE CALORIES

- *Choose something you enjoy doing or you'll never keep it up! Think back to activities you've enjoyed in the past and try something similar – for example, if you enjoyed team sports, join a netball or football team, or if you enjoy dancing, try a choreographed fitness or dance class.*
- *Exercise with a partner or friend. They'll give you moral support and motivate you to keep going when you don't feel like it. Research shows that 90 per cent of us prefer to exercise with others, and we are up to 22 per cent more likely to continue if we exercise with other people.*
- *Set yourself realistic goals which you can achieve over approximately six weeks. Good examples include building up to run a specific distance, doing a set number of exercise classes, or completing a specific number of minutes of exercise.*

HOW MUCH EFFORT DO I HAVE TO PUT IN?

Most of us exercise well within our comfort zone, at a level that feels comfortable, without getting out of breath or sweating too much. However, this fails to give us a 'training effect'. On a scale of 1–10 of the rate of perceived exertion (RPE), we often remain below 5. To really make a difference, you should exercise at a perceived exertion rate of 7–8. You should feel slightly out of breath, and be able to speak a sentence but not have a conversation!

HOW LONG SHOULD I EXERCISE FOR?

The longer you exercise for, the more calories you will use up. As we use up stored carbohydrate, we begin to use more fat, so exercising for longer results in more fat being used up. For exercise sessions longer than 40 minutes duration, you should work out at a medium intensity of about 6 or 7 RPE to maximize fat-burning potential.

If you have less than 40 minutes available for a workout, you will need to exercise at a higher intensity for the same caloric expenditure. Try to exercise at a RPE of 8.

Insight
Weight-bearing exercises such as walking, running or aerobic fitness classes will use more calories than seated exercises such as rowing or cycling at the same intensity and duration. This is because you are carrying your body weight at the same time as exercising.

WHAT IF I CAN'T FIND TIME TO EXERCISE?

Remember, every bit counts, even if you only exercise for 20 minutes, it might use up an extra 100 calories. Three of these shorter workouts each week can help you to lose an extra pound of fat over 12 weeks, on top of weight loss resulting from other exercise and reduced calorie intake.

WHAT ABOUT WEIGHT TRAINING ... WON'T IT MAKE ME GAIN WEIGHT?

Weight training is an effective way to increase lean tissue. You won't build large muscles unless you follow a body building routine. Two sessions of weight training weekly will really make a difference to your body shape and weight loss, as the extra lean tissue increases your metabolic rate, unlike body fat. Extra muscle may make you weigh a little heavier initially, but this helps you to use up more calories, and you will soon notice a reduction in clothes sizes and measurements.

Insight: The best exercise for weight loss

Interval training is very effective for weight loss – this is when you work hard for a minute then exercise at a lower intensity for a minute (you can alter the timings). It enables you to exercise at a higher intensity than you usually would, as you only stay at this level for a short period of time. During the higher intensity phase you use up more calories than normal.

3 Eating less and exercising more

If you're really keen to lose weight, reducing your calorie intake and increasing your calorie expenditure will obviously create a bigger calorie deficit, as you take in less and use up more energy. Just make sure you're eating enough to provide energy for your exercise sessions!

Insight: Change the way you think about dieting

A little bit of what you fancy does you good, as long as it is a little bit, and not too often! We often struggle with weight maintenance because the extra mouthful, the stolen chip, or the forgotten biscuit all add up. Change your way of thinking so that instead of convincing yourself that the extra mouthful won't matter, understand that leaving a little on your plate will make a difference, because over a week, a month and certainly a year, a few extra calories here and there do add up to extra weight.

Seven-day eating plan for healthy weight loss

Day 1

Breakfast	Porridge made with soya milk. Add linseeds, red grapes, cherries.
Mid-morning	Mixed fruit salad with berries, mango, apricots and red grapes.
Lunch	Tomato soup with rice cakes and a small salad with garlic and onion.
Dinner	Baked salmon steak with broccoli, cauliflower and baked sweet potato.

Day 2

Breakfast	Soy yoghurt with berries and linseeds.
Mid-morning	Celery, carrot and pepper crudités with cherry tomatoes and rice cakes.
Lunch	Mixed bean salad with chick peas and brown rice, tomatoes, garlic, onions, cucumber, radish, celery and tomatoes.
Dinner	Brown rice with garlic-roasted root vegetables, fennel and broccoli.

Day 3

Breakfast	Mixed fruit salad with berries, mango, apricots and red grapes.
Mid-morning	Oat-based sugar-free cereal bar and fresh fruit.
Lunch	Sardines with brown rice and mixed bean salad and salad vegetables.
Dinner	Savoy cabbage/red onion stir fry with added vegetables including fennel.

Day 4

Breakfast	Porridge or millet made with soya milk with added linseeds and berries.
Mid-morning	Rice cakes with tomatoes, raw carrot and raw pepper crudités.
Lunch	Mackerel served on oatcakes or rice cakes with salad vegetables.
Dinner	Brown rice vegetable risotto including garlic, onion, cress and tomatoes.

Day 5

Breakfast	Mixed fruit salad with berries, mango, apricots, peach and red grapes.
Mid-morning	Soy yoghurt sprinkled with linseeds and rice cakes.
Lunch	Baked potato with beans and a mixed salad.
Dinner	Bean and vegetable curry, chilli or stew with steamed brown rice.

Day 6

Breakfast	Millet made with soya milk with added linseeds and berries.
Snacks	Tomatoes, raw peppers and carrot crudités with rice cakes.
Lunch	Lentil soup (no salt) with rice cakes.
Dinner	Steamed fish with garlic-roasted squash, fennel, sweet potato and broccoli.

Day 7

Breakfast	Mixed fruit salad with berries, mango, apricots, peach and red grapes.
Mid-morning	Rice cakes with raw carrot and broccoli, tomatoes and raw peppers.
Lunch	Roast Sunday dinner (with very little gravy and no/little meat).
Dinner	Watercress soup and oat cakes.

THINGS TO REMEMBER

Ten commandments for weight-loss success:

- *Eat slowly, and once you feel full, stop eating! If your plate is still half full, your portion was too large. By leaving just a couple of mouthfuls on the plate, you consume fewer calories and get used to smaller portions, allowing your stomach size to reduce. It will feel uncomfortable if you begin to eat larger portions again.*

- *Very often we mistake thirst for hunger pangs. If you feel like a snack, drink a glass of water and wait for ten minutes to see if the temptation to snack disappears.*

- *It's important to make small changes towards a healthier diet for life. Many people feel that being on a diet is an 'all or nothing' regime, and feel like they have failed if they over-indulge. Occasional over-indulgences are part of life and do not make or break a life-long healthy eating plan.*

- *Over-indulged at the weekend? Have a couple of healthy days with plenty of exercise, no alcohol or high-fat/high-sugar foods to offset the damage and re-balance the scales. However, use this as an occasional remedy, as the body does prefer a more even keel!*

- *Losing any type of body weight other than body fat is counterproductive. Water loss leaves you dehydrated and the weight returns as soon as you drink fluids; losing lean tissue reduces your metabolism, reducing the rate at which you use up calories; reduced weight from lower carbohydrate intake returns as soon as you consume carbohydrates again.*

- *Weight loss is quicker when you have more body fat to lose. Your body automatically uses more fat for energy, and the more you weigh, the more energy it takes to move around. This explains the typical weight-loss plateau that may occur after a few weeks. Remember – you'll need fewer calories for weight maintenance once you weigh less.*

* *Using tape measurements or feeling how comfortably clothes fit are both effective alternative ways of monitoring weight loss.*

* *If you reduce your calorie intake below your Basal Metabolic Rate you may slow down your metabolism, and weight loss will become slower and more difficult. Very low-calorie diets are therefore counterproductive to losing weight.*

* *The most effective way to lose body fat is through a combination of healthy eating and regular exercise.*

* *Regular eating is essential for success: breakfast increases your metabolism in the morning and helps you to avoid mid-morning munchies; eating regularly keeps your metabolism high, and avoids low blood sugar levels which promote snacking; missing meals leads to high-calorie foods and over-eating at the next meal; eating smaller amounts throughout the day allows you to make more use of what you have eaten, and store less.*

3

....

Superfoods

In this chapter you will learn:
- *what the best superfoods are*
- *how superfoods enhance your health*
- *simple ways to get superfoods into your diet.*

It can be difficult to eat a healthy diet if you have a busy lifestyle, lack of time or a food-fussy family! However, if you want to make the most of the time and food readily available to you with minimum effort and maximum reward, then read on. Nutrient-dense superfoods are lurking on supermarket shelves, in your fridge, even in your garden and, with a little bit of know-how, a superfood diet can be as easy as your normal eating habits.

Start right now!

1 *Eat something naturally orange and green every day.*
2 *Buy spinach, rocket or watercress instead of cos or iceberg lettuce.*
3 *Add berries to your breakfast cereal.*

DONE!

What are superfoods?

Superfoods are foods which go above and beyond providing just calories and the usual range of vitamins and minerals and are either exceptionally rich in specific nutrients or contain compounds which bestow health benefits. These compounds sometimes belong to a 'family' or group of nutrients which have been proven to enhance health or help to fight disease, such as the carotenoids. Many so-called 'superfoods' contain phytonutrients (plant nutrients), which are compounds that have not yet been proven as essential in the diet, but are known to offer health benefits.

Phytonutrients

HOW DO PHYTONUTRIENTS WORK?

Phytonutrients enhance our health in many different ways, but there are two major ways in which they work:

- As *anti-oxidants*.
- As *enzyme-inducers*.

Anti-oxidants
Anti-oxidants 'quench' free radicals in our body, which can stop cellular damage from occurring. This may mean slowing down skin ageing, reducing inflammation, or even offering additional protection against diseases such as heart disease or cancer (see Chapter 6 for more information on anti-ageing foods).

Enzyme-inducers
We need a number of different nutrients to feed our enzyme systems and this is especially important in the liver where most detoxification takes place. Some of these foods earn their superfood status by providing the nutrients required for detoxification or inducing our enzyme systems to carry out this vital role.

Although superfoods can be any sort of foods, many nutrients are found in vegetables and fruits alone, and these are collectively known as phytonutrients (phyto means plant).

PHYTONUTRIENT FOOD FAMILIES

Flavonoids

This group of compounds has been shown to have anti-allergic, anti-bacterial, anti-oxidant and anti-inflammatory properties. They convey anti-tumour benefits as well as providing cardio-protective elements which counteract heart disease. There are several sub-groups within the flavonoid 'family', the most common are shown in Table 8 with examples of the foods that contain them. The foods richest in flavonoids include onions and apples, and they are also found in red wine and tea. You'll learn more about some of these nutrients and foods later on in this chapter and throughout the book.

Get your flavonoid fix now!

For a superfood berry smoothie, try blending one cup of berries (any type) with one ripe banana and a cup of soya milk.

DONE!

Check that the foods in Table 8 are on your shopping list so that you can follow the seven-day superfood eating plan at the end of this chapter. In the meantime, make sure you include at least three flavonoid foods in your daily diet:

- ✓ *Include onions in either lunch or dinner.*
- ✓ *Eat an apple a day.*
- ✓ *Swap your usual brew for green tea.*

Flavonoid family

Flavonoid family	Examples of foods
Anthocyanins and Pro-anthocyanidins	Grape seeds
	Red grapes and berries
	Plums and prunes
	Red apples
	Aubergines
	Red wine
Flavonols	Onions
	Parsley
	Kale
Isoflavonoids	Oranges, lemons and limes
	Grapefruit
	Apples
Catechins	Green tea
Isoflavones	Soya beans, kidney beans, lima beans and mung beans

Carotenoids

The carotenoids are usually easy to spot, as they are found in foods that are naturally red, orange or yellow in colour. They are also found in dark green vegetables, but the orange pigment is hidden by the green pigment found in the chlorophyll present in green vegetables.

Insight: Add carotenoids to your cooking!

Some carotenoids become more available during digestion if the foods containing them are cooked ... a great example is lycopene found in tomatoes. Use tinned tomatoes for a quick pasta sauce or a base for curries and casseroles.

Carotenoids have been proven to have anti-cancer properties. Their anti-oxidant nature supports immune function, and also reduces the risk of macular degeneration (impaired vision which can lead to blindness) and cataracts, making this group of foods essential for better eye health. The carotenoids consist of different types of compounds, some of which are listed below.

Carotenoids

Beta carotene	Found in carrots, sweet potato, pumpkin and other orange-coloured fruits and vegetables such as apricots.
Lutein and Zeaxanthin	Found in green and yellow fruits and vegetables such as cabbage, green beans, avocado or honeydew melon. Also found in orange-coloured foods.
Lycopene	Found in high levels in tomatoes, and in tomato products (for example, purée).

For a carotenoid-rich diet add these foods to your shopping list so that you can follow the seven-day superfoods eating plan in this chapter.

Add these carotenoid-rich foods to your shopping list now:

▸ *carrots*
▸ *sweet potato*
▸ *squash or pumpkin*
▸ *red, orange or yellow peppers or capsicums*
▸ *sweetcorn*
▸ *fresh and tinned tomatoes*
▸ *a selection of spinach, watercress and rocket*
▸ *broccoli and cabbage*
▸ *a selection of papaya, mango, cantaloupe melon, nectarines, peaches, apricots and pineapple*
▸ *fresh parsley.*

Sulphur compounds
This group of phytonutrients is split into several different compounds, but the main classifications are the indoles and the isothiocyanates. These compounds induce enzyme activity, supporting the detoxification processes in the liver (see Chapter 4).

Many of the indoles are found in Brassica vegetables which include broccoli, cabbage (including red cabbage), red-leaved lettuce, kale, cauliflower and sprouts. Other foods containing sulphur compounds include radishes, onions and garlic. Garlic is listed as a superfood in its own right due to the incredible wealth of health benefits it offers – more about that later!

Cholesterol-lowering compounds

Phytosterols are similar to the cholesterol found in animal foods such as the egg yolk, but are the plant derivative, hence the name phytosterols. However, rather than raise our cholesterol levels, the phytosterols do the opposite – they help to lower cholesterol. Phytosterols naturally occur in a range of plant foods, and are found mostly in vegetable oils. It is these compounds – plant sterols and stannols – that are added to foods such as yoghurts or margarines to help lower cholesterol, making them 'functional foods' (see Chapter 5 for more information).

Phytosterols compete with cholesterol for absorption in the digestive tract, blocking the amount of dietary cholesterol that can be absorbed. They also inhibit the re-absorption of cholesterol from bile acids during the digestive process, again reducing the amount of cholesterol entering the bloodstream.

Most carbohydrate foods contain some fibre which will help to lower cholesterol, for example, oats are effective in cholesterol-lowering diets, the beta glucan fibre in oats being the active ingredient. However, there are certain types of fibre, inulin, for example, which are really effective at carrying cholesterol out of the body. Inulin is found in foods such as garlic, onion, asparagus, Jerusalem artichoke and chicory.

The cholesterol in our bloodstream comes from two sources – cholesterol that we consume in foods such as egg yolks, and the cholesterol that our liver makes. Some of the cholesterol we make is carried, via the bile, into the small intestine during food digestion, when fibre such as inulin can absorb some of this cholesterol and carry it out of the body in the faeces.

The essential fatty acids

No list of superfoods would be complete without those rich in the essential fatty acids. Although we need both types of essential fatty acid, most people eat enough of the omega 6 type, but lack omega 3 fats in their diet. Check out the lists below to see if you're eating enough omega 6 and omega 3 fats.

Foods rich in omega 3	*Foods rich in omega 6*
Oily fish	Margarines
Linseeds (flaxseeds)	Vegetable oils
Walnuts	Nuts and seeds

Most seeds and nuts contain both types of fat, but usually contain more of the omega 6 fats. Although the omega 6 and omega 3 groups of fatty acids include several different fats, each group contains an essential fatty acid that we need in our diet:

linoleic acid (omega 6) and linolenic acid (omega 3).

Although many foods contain omega 3 and omega 6 fatty acids, very few have a healthy omega 6: omega 3 ratio, so over time, many people have an unbalanced fatty acid intake as shown below:

Normal healthy ratio   3:1 (omega 6:omega 3)
Typical western diet ratio   16–20:1 (omega 6:omega 3)

Therefore, after following such a diet for a number of years, many of us need a ratio that is strongly in favour of the omega 3 fats to correct an imbalance.

As both types of fatty acids affect our inflammatory pathways, if we have too much of one type of fat and not enough of the other, we often experience inflammatory symptoms:

- *hay fever*
- *asthma*
- *eczema*
- *psoriasis*
- *arthritis.*

We need lots of different nutrients to ensure that these pathways are effective, but consuming a correct ratio of essential fatty acids in your diet is a good place to start. It's worth doing as well, as the essential fatty acids affect much more than our inflammatory pathways …

Tips for a healthy heart
- *Essential fatty acids affect the integrity and flexibility of our arteries, contributing to hypertension and atherosclerosis when the balance isn't right.*
- *Foods rich in saturated fat and cholesterol often contain poor levels of omega 3 fats, which not only make the arterial walls less flexible, but add to the risk of fatty plaques in the arteries.*

- *In comparison, the essential fatty acids and long chain fish oils keep the artery walls flexible, limiting arterial damage and reducing the risk of heart disease.*
- *Polyunsaturated fats also help to reduce cholesterol levels, high levels of which contribute to heart disease.*

Insight: Does fish make you brainy?

Fish contains types of omega 3 fatty acids that are essential for healthy brain function – this explains the link between fish and improved memory and enhanced mental function.

WHAT IF YOU DON'T EAT FISH?

Don't worry, all is not lost. Linolenic acid, the omega 3 fatty acid found in linseeds, linseed oil and walnuts, can be converted into the longer chain polyunsaturated fatty acids normally found in fish, although the conversion rate may be very low – less than one per cent. Here are some fish-free strategies …

Insight: Long chain fatty acids in a fish-free zone

- *Add linseeds to yoghurts, cereals, smoothies, salads and stir fries.*
- *Use linseed oil as a salad dressing.*
- *Use rapeseed oil as a salad dressing or for stir fries.*
- *Snack on walnuts.*

So, a picture of the perfect diet is beginning to form:

1 *Eat a naturally colourful diet with plenty of purple, red, green, orange and yellow fruits and vegetables.*
2 *Add some oily fish, oils and seeds for essential fatty acids.*
3 *Cook with garlic and onions.*

There, you have the beginnings of a naturally healthy, superfood diet!

However, there are some foods which have numerous health-promoting properties which make them stand out from other foods and merit being eaten every day.

Jackie has followed a superfoods diet for several
years – it takes no extra time or effort, she enjoys the
foods and especially enjoys the comments on her age,
'Everyone I meet thinks I look at least ten years younger
than I actually am – I know I have my diet to thank
for that.'

Meet the superfoods

ONIONS (WHITE, RED, SHALLOTS, SPRING ... ANY TYPE)

Onions contain a phytonutrient called quercetin, which belongs to
the flavonoid family. Flavonoids have so many health benefits they
are sometimes referred to as 'vitamin P'.

Major flavonoid benefits

▶ *Anti-histamine*
▶ *Anti-viral*
▶ *Anti-bacterial*
▶ *Anti-inflammatory*
▶ *Anti-allergic.*

Eat at least one medium-sized onion every day if you suffer with
arthritis, irritable bowel syndrome, inflammatory skin conditions,
or allergies such as hay fever or asthma.

GARLIC

Both onion and garlic were used in ancient Egypt, Greece and Italy for heart disease. Garlic contains a number of sulphur compounds which provide its pungent odour but are also extremely beneficial for our health.

Major garlic benefits

- ▶ *Anti-bacterial*
- ▶ *Anti-viral*
- ▶ *Anti-fungal*
- ▶ *Anti-thrombotic*
- ▶ *Anti-carcinogenic.*

Insight: How garlic helps you have a healthy heart

- ▶ *It 'thins' the blood, making it less likely to clot.*
- ▶ *It reduces 'bad' low-density lipoprotein (LDL) cholesterol and triglycerides (fats) in the blood.*
- ▶ *It contains inulin fibre which helps to reduce cholesterol.*

In addition to keeping our cardiovascular system healthy, garlic has a number of other benefits. The inulin acts as a prebiotic to help promote healthy bowel flora or 'good' bacteria (see more on this in Chapter 5). Together with its anti-microbial, anti-fungal properties, which can reduce the risk of bacterial or yeast infections, including garlic in your diet every day will contribute to improved cardiovascular, immune and bowel health.

For allicin, the active ingredient of garlic, to be most active, it should not be heated, so grated raw garlic will be more effective than including it in your cooking. However, simply including garlic in your cooking will still offer several health benefits – see the seven-day superfood eating plan and recipes to see how easy it is to include in your diet.

Although garlic capsules are less pungent, it is unknown whether all the health benefits are still present after this amount of processing. As with all foods and nutrients, fresh is generally best!

CRUCIFEROUS/BRASSICA VEGETABLES (BROCCOLI, CAULIFLOWER, SPROUTS, CABBAGE)

This group of vegetables contains phytonutrients called indoles and isothiocyanates. These compounds are powerful detoxifying nutrients, and have been linked to reduced incidences of cancer. The younger sprouts are more potent, but all these vegetables – ideally organically grown – should be used freely in the diet.

Major benefits of dark green leafy vegetables

▶ *These vegetables are rich sources of calcium, magnesium, potassium, iron and vitamin C.*
▶ *They also contain the carotenoids beta carotene and lutein, which support eye health, and have also been proven to have anti-tumour properties in some types of malignancies such as lung cancer and breast cancer. Lutein is also found in green beans, avocado, peppers, apricots and pumpkin.*

TOMATOES (LYCOPENE)

Much has been written about the benefits of a tomato-rich diet for its super-nutrient lycopene, which has been shown to reduce the incidence of breast and prostate cancers. Although fresh (organic) tomatoes should always be included in your weekly shopping list, the lycopene is still available in tomato soup, pastes and purées and even in tinned tomatoes.

> **Inisight**
> Try to include tomatoes in your diet every day. Research has shown that availability of the nutrients locked into the tomato increases with cooking, so go ahead and enjoy roasted tomatoes, tomato soups and tapenades, tomato-based chillies and curries!

CAROTENE-RICH FRUIT AND VEGETABLES (ORANGE, YELLOW, RED IN COLOUR)

There is overwhelming evidence that vegetables rich in beta-carotene have an anti-carcinogenic effect. Beta-carotene is the super-nutrient found mostly in vegetables of a yellow to orange colour. Dark green vegetables are also rich in beta-carotene, but other pigments hide the familiar beta-carotene colour.

What does beta carotene do?

▶ *It contributes to a healthy immune system.*
▶ *Helps to protect against some eye diseases such as macular degeneration.*
▶ *It offers anti-oxidant benefits for better overall health and longevity.*

BERRIES, CHERRIES AND GRAPES

Another important group of nutrients is the proanthocyanidins, found in abundance in dark red or purple fruits and vegetables such as red grapes (even some red wines – more about that in Chapter 6), cherries and berries. These compounds have anti-ageing and disease preventive properties through their anti-oxidant activity, and have been linked with combating atherosclerosis (furring of the arteries in coronary heart disease), joint disease and cancer.

Insight

One of the richest sources of proanthocyanidins is
the grape seed, so swap seedless white grapes for red ones
with the seed, and crunch away! Grape seed extract is
commonly added to skin creams and lotions in the hope
that the anti-oxidants will prevent some of the free radical
damage which causes wrinkles and skin ageing. If you don't
fancy crunching on grape seeds, grape seed supplements are
readily available.

ORGANIC, OILY FISH (SALMON, TROUT, SARDINES, MACKEREL, PILCHARDS)

Not all superfoods are from the plant kingdom! Oily fish are
rich in two types of omega 3 fatty acids – eicosapentanoic acid
(EPA) and docosahexanoic acid (DHA). These long chain fatty
acids are used to form 'insulating' membranes around the nerves,
enabling messages to be transferred in the brain and nervous
system.

Foods rich in EPA and DHA
Salmon, mackerel, pilchards, sardines, tuna, herring.

Insight

If you don't like fish, take a fish oil supplement.
There are even special fish oil supplements for children
following a significant amount of research illustrating
improvements in conditions such as hyperactivity, dyslexia
and autism.

At the other end of the age range, a sufficient supply of
long chain fatty acids can improve conditions such as
senile dementia. Because they also have anti-inflammatory
properties, fish and fish oil supplements are commonly
included in therapeutic diets for arthritis, allergies and
inflammatory health conditions.

Did you know?

White fish such as cod or haddock do contain EPA and DHA, but as they store fat in their liver rather than in their flesh, you have to consume cod liver oil capsules to get the fish oils. Although oily fish store fat in their flesh, the essential oils are mostly lost during the canning process, so tinned fish will contain reduced levels of fatty acids similar to the levels found in non-oily fish.

Non-fish alternatives

Remember, if you don't eat fish you can convert alpha-linolenic acid, an essential fatty acid, into the longer polyunsaturated fatty acid chains normally found in fish, but you'd have to be filling up on linseeds (flaxseed), walnuts, linseed or rapeseed oil. If these foods aren't a mainstay of your diet, a fish oil supplement may be an option for you, as only small amounts of alpha-linolenic acid can be lengthened into EPA or DHA. Check out the best nuts, seeds and oils in Table 10 if you don't eat fish.

The linolenic acid (omega 3) content in nuts, seeds and oils

	Omega 3 (g/100 g)	Omega 6 (g/100 g)
Linseed/linseed oil	51.5	13
Walnut	7	3.6
Brazil nut	0	23.5
Almonds	0.3	10
Sunflower seeds	0.14	24.6
Sunflower oil	0.27	46.8
Olive oil	0.6	9.9

SEEDS AND SEED OILS

As well as providing the essential fatty acids, seeds are a wonder of nature, providing an abundance of vitamins and minerals alongside a good fibre intake. Pumpkin seeds, for example, are rich in zinc and should be included in the diet of any non-meat eaters. If you like nuts, you'll probably enjoy eating seeds, but here are some ideas on how to include seeds in your diet.

Insight: Feeding seeds to your body

- *Make up your own seed mix to add to cereals, yoghurts and stir fries – try a mix of pumpkin, sunflower, sesame and linseed.*
- *Try bars with added seeds such as the '9 bar' with linseeds and chocolate … who said healthy eating couldn't be tasty?*
- *Buy tubs of seeds to nibble on at your desk or in the evening, some are roasted or have herbs and spices such as chilli added – check out the FOOD DOCTOR range for a tasty treat.*

You really are what you eat

Our body fat is made up of the type of fatty acids we commonly eat, so if you have eaten very little oily fish or seeds rich in linolenic acid over a number of years, your body fat will contain an unbalanced ratio of fatty acids. Whenever you break down your body fat for energy, the fatty acids are released into the bloodstream, so don't expect to correct a fatty acid imbalance overnight … remember, you are what you eat – literally! If you think this applies to you, avoid sunflower seeds for the first few months of your seed-fest, as these seeds contain much more omega 6 than omega 3 fatty acids and will slow down your efforts to correct your fatty acid imbalance.

SOYA BEANS

Soya beans contain isoflavones, a type of flavonoid. The isoflavone content decreases severely with processing into soya milk or tofu, but soya products are still a worthy addition to your diet.

Major soya benefits

▶ *Soya has anti-cancer and anti-oxidant properties as a flavonoid.*
▶ *It has also been proven to help reduce cholesterol levels.*
▶ *The isoflavones in soya beans may alleviate menopausal problems such as hot flushes and osteoporosis – this is because isoflavones are phyto-oestrogens (plant oestrogens).*

Phyto-oestrogens have a subtle oestrogenic effect in the body: they attach to the oestrogen receptors on our cells, exerting a milder oestrogenic effect than oestrogen. In this way, these foods reduce the normal oestrogenic effect that oestrogen has, as some of the cell receptors are already 'blocked' by phyto-oestrogens. Several foods contain phyto-oestrogens, although the soya bean has the richest content. As the active isoflavones in soya exert a hormonal effect, it is safer to simply consume soya products as part of a healthy, balanced diet rather than take concentrated supplements.

Phyto-oestrogenic foods

Apples, yams, cherries, coconuts, plums, potatoes, peppers, aubergine, tomatoes, olives, carrots, wheat germ.

GREEN TEA

Tea varieties include white, black, green and oolong, although black tea is mostly consumed in the west, whilst Asian countries such as Japan, China and India favour green tea. The teas are manufactured in similar ways, but oxidation is prevented in green tea leaves, increasing the levels of health-promoting polyphenolic compounds called catechins.

Health benefits of catechins

▶ *They help to control inflammation and cell growth, promoting anti-tumour properties.*
▶ *Catechins are powerful anti-oxidants, which help to reduce free radical damage in the body.*
▶ *They support the immune system and improve cell function.*

As with grape seeds, green tea is another product often found in skin preparations due to its anti-oxidant and anti-inflammatory properties; hence it can be used both topically and in the diet.

Insight: Beauty tip

Green tea has been proven to promote health when drunk and when applied to the skin. To enjoy the benefits of both, freeze some freshly brewed green tea as ice cubes and each morning allow one to defrost onto a cotton wool pad. Use the liquid as a toner, or apply to the skin under moisturizer or sun cream for additional anti-oxidant, anti-ageing benefits.

And another thing ...

The catechins found in green tea have been found to support pancreatic function, in particular, the cells responsible for the production of insulin which helps to regulate blood sugar levels. According to legend, in 2737BC the Chinese Emperor Shen-Nung discovered green tea and it has been used in China as a remedy for diabetes and other ailments since. Between two and ten tea infusions daily is recommended to enjoy the benefits of green tea, so get brewing!

TURMERIC

Curcumin is the natural yellow colouring in the spice turmeric. It stands out as a superfood because of its anti-mutagenic and anti-cancer properties which it exerts through enhancing detoxification in the liver. It has anti-oxidant properties and prevents oxidation of fats such as cholesterol in the body.

Spice up your life!

Use turmeric freely in soups, dressings, marinades, curries and sauces – include it in any way that you can to get a useful teaspoonful included in your daily diet.

Simple tips for increasing your superfood intake

So now you know which foods earn 'superfood' status, the next thing is to plan how to include these foods in your diet. It can be as easy as choosing spinach over iceberg lettuce at the supermarket! Read on for tips that will help you to create a superfood diet.

GO GREEN

When choosing salad leaves, always opt for the dark green leaves such as spinach, rocket or watercress. Paler leaves such as cos or iceberg lettuce provide mostly fibre and water, and don't contain the same levels of vitamins, minerals or phytonutrients as the darker leaves. Check out the comparison below...

Nutrient levels of salad leaves

Nutrient (mg/100 g) unless stated otherwise	Spinach (raw)	Iceberg lettuce
Magnesium	54	5
Calcium	170	19
Potassium	500	160

Vitamin C	26	3
Iron	2.1	0.4
Carotene (mcg)	3535	50
Vitamin E	1.71	0.57

(Figures taken from McCance and Widdowson's *The Composition of Foods*, 6th Ed.)

ADD A LITTLE EXTRA SPICE

Herbs and spices have been used for centuries for their medicinal and health properties and by adding a herb or spice to your meal you will enhance the flavour and presentation whilst simultaneously boosting your nutrient intake. Many herbs and spices contain health-promoting active compounds, the green leafy herbs such as parsley also providing good levels of carotenes and vitamin C. This is how easy it can be:

▶ *Add a generous sprinkle of coriander to yoghurt, fish or curry-based sauces and soups.*
▶ *Add a spoonful of chopped chilli to dressings, salads and stir fries.*
▶ *Use basil for tomato or pasta dishes, or sprinkle over Mediterranean-inspired salads with avocado, vine-ripened tomatoes and olive oil. Don't forget a generous handful on your freshly-made tomato soup!*
▶ *Add a handful of freshly chopped chilli, coriander, basil or parsley to shop-bought soups, sauces, salads or dips to boost the nutrient content and taste of your convenience meal.*
▶ *Add a pinch of cinnamon or turmeric to porridge.*
▶ *Use turmeric in curries, casseroles and stews, or as a base for a salad dressing.*

If you find buying fresh herbs expensive, why not start your own herb garden? You can grow a variety of herbs in a small garden plot, in planters in the yard or on a roof terrace, or even in plant pots on your window sill. This can give the rest of the family (especially children) a healthy appreciation for fresh food. If the herbs are picked straight from the stem you're guaranteed a higher nutrient content and the medicinal benefits that are no longer present in dried herbs. See Chapter 9 for tips on growing your own.

HEALTHY HABITS

Get into the habit of using nutrient-rich foods on a regular basis – in fact, try to add at least one superfood to every meal. Here's a few ways of boosting your nutrient intake.

- ▶ *Add brightly coloured fruit to breakfast cereals, and onions, tomatoes, peppers or spinach to cooked breakfasts.*
- ▶ *Get into the habit of always adding salad vegetables to sandwiches, with grated carrot, beetroot, tomato, dark green leaves and onions always stocked in the fridge.*
- ▶ *Spinach, watercress or rocket can be added to most meals – wilt into risottos or pasta dishes, serve on the side drizzled with an olive or seed oil, garlic and chilli dressing, or add with grated beetroot to favourite snacks such as sardines on toast or filled bagels.*
- ▶ *Onions and garlic make a great start for any stir fries, casseroles or soups – make these your starting point in any dish.*
- ▶ *Top up the fridge and fruit bowl with superfoods to snack on: red grapes, cherries, carrot or pepper crudités, mangoes and papayas – all ready to eat or blend.*

Brighten up your dishes
Vegetables and fruits that are naturally yellow, orange or red in colour will contain high levels of beta carotene, a natural anti-oxidant. Plan meals that always include something bright on your plate. Here are some ideas:

Breakfasts:

- ▶ *Superfood fruit salad – apricot, red grapes, blueberries, strawberries, raspberries, kiwi, water melon and pineapple.*
- ▶ *Add chopped apple, berries or mango to breakfast cereals.*
- ▶ *Include at least one brightly coloured fruit in a breakfast smoothie.*

Lunches:

- ▶ *Superfood salad – dark green leaves, beetroot, carrot, onion, red grapes, avocado, tomatoes (raw or roasted in olive oil), drizzled with a linseed oil, chilli and grated garlic dressing.*
- ▶ *Superfood soups – made from fresh with a base of onion and garlic with olive oil, then choose your main ingredient from tomatoes, squash, sweet potato, carrot or watercress. Add chillies for a spicy kick, turmeric for healthy colour, or lentils for a more sustaining soup.*

Dinners:

- ▶ *Superfood risotto – add roasted sweet potato or squash and rocket.*
- ▶ *Superfood pasta – add fresh, tinned or roasted tomatoes, red onions, aubergines (eggplant) and basil for a healthy Mediterranean-inspired dish.*
- ▶ *Stuff yellow, orange or red peppers with stir fried onion, garlic, sweet corn, chopped tomatoes and baked sweet potato mix, then bake!*

Old favourites
Make a baked potato a healthier option by baking a sweet potato instead and adding a superfood salad. If eggs are on the menu, add peppers, onions, garlic, spinach and tomatoes to an omelette; serve scrambled or poached eggs on a bed of spinach.

Store cupboard basics
It all starts with the shopping – if you haven't got these foods in the house, they won't be eaten! Make sure that these foods are on your shopping list every week: Onions, garlic, spinach, rocket, watercress, broccoli, cabbage, cauliflower, carrots, beetroot, tomatoes, sweet potato, squash, berries, red grapes, cherries, mangoes, papaya, apricots, nectarines, apples, peppers, avocado, oily fish, linseeds, pumpkin and sunflower seeds, nuts, green tea and soya products such as soya milk and soya beans.

Add other superfoods to your shopping list as and when you need them to create superfood recipes and meals ... chillies, turmeric, coriander ...

So, now you know which foods to include for enhanced good health, you've made your shopping list, and have some ideas for superfood meals. Here's an idea of what a seven-day superfood eating plan could look like ... maybe healthy eating is not so difficult after all!

Superfoods seven-day eating plan

Day 1

Breakfast — Mixed berry smoothie made with blueberries, strawberries and raspberries, live yoghurt, a teaspoon of linseed oil or linseeds mixed with mineral water or soya or oat milk.

Lunch — Sardines on wholemeal toast with a large green salad, tomatoes, beetroot, grated carrot, grated garlic and red onion.

Dinner — Stuffed baked vegetables (see recipe, page 88).

Day 2

Breakfast — Superfood fruit salad – mango, papaya, apricots, cantaloupe melon, red cherries, red grapes, kiwi and mixed berries. Serve with live Greek yoghurt and a sprinkle of flaked almonds and mixed seeds.

Lunch — Freshly made tomato soup with a sprinkle of red chillies and freshly chopped herbs (see recipe, page 85).

Dinner — Seared tuna or salmon steak with mushrooms, garlic and shallots, served with a baked sweet potato and lightly steamed broccoli (see recipe, page 87).

Day 3

Breakfast   Porridge with soya or oat milk topped with mixed
             berries and mixed seeds.

Lunch   Poached, tinned or smoked salmon with mixed salad
             vegetables: watercress, rocket, tomatoes, beetroot,
             red onions, radishes, grated carrot and bean sprouts.
             Serve with a salad dressing of linseed or rapeseed oil,
             turmeric, chopped garlic and fresh lemon juice.

Dinner   Savoy (spring) cabbage stir fry with red onions,
             garlic, mushrooms, sweetcorn, fresh peppers
             and mixed seeds. Stir fry and add tofu (see recipe,
             page 86).

Day 4

Breakfast   Soya or live yoghurt topped with half a banana and
             berries, and a spoonful of mixed seeds and nuts.

Lunch   Freshly made pumpkin soup with a diced red chilli
             and fresh coriander sprinkled on top.

Dinner   Organically reared game (pheasant, partridge) if
             meat is eaten. If not, choose organic fresh fish. Serve
             with garlic-roasted carrots, sweet potato, shallots
             and parsnip, and lightly steamed cauliflower or
             broccoli.

Day 5

Breakfast   Fresh fruit juice – your choice of blended blueberries,
             strawberries and raspberries, or juiced organic apple
             and carrot. Add a teaspoon of linseed oil or linseeds
             to your juice. A spoonful of live yoghurt and an
             optional banana will turn your juice into a more
             substantial smoothie.

Lunch   Mixed bean salad. Add mixed beans and chick
             peas to a salad of freshly grated carrot, garlic and
             beetroot, rocket leaves, radishes and tomatoes. Add
             linseed oil with chopped chillies as a salad dressing
             and dress with fresh herbs.

Dinner   Salmon, sweet potato and rocket risotto (see recipe,
             page 86).

Day 6

Breakfast	Granola served with soya or oat milk, live yoghurt and fresh fruit (see recipe in Chapter 9, page 252).
Lunch	Spanish omelette with onions, garlic, chopped peppers and tomatoes. Serve with a large green salad and grated beetroot.
Dinner	Sweet potato curry with brown rice (see recipe, below).

Day 7

Breakfast	Sunday morning kedgeree (see recipe, page 85).
Lunch	Watercress and broccoli soup topped with freshly grated carrot and beetroot.
Dinner	Baked organic salmon or trout served with baby carrots, Savoy cabbage strips and sweet potato wedges dusted in turmeric and roasted in a little olive oil with garlic.

Superfood recipes

Follow these simple recipes to help you enjoy the superfoods seven-day eating plan. Even if these meals are quite different to your usual cooking habits, once you've made them a couple of times, they'll be as quick and easy as any meal – but with twice the amount of nutrients! There are also a couple of extra recipes for you to try.

Superfood curry

Ingredients for 2 people

1 tbs olive oil
1 small tin chick peas
1 large sweet potato or squash
200 g fresh tomatoes
3 large tbs Greek yoghurt
2 large carrots
1 onion
2 cloves garlic
2 tsps turmeric

Handful fresh coriander
2 red chillies, chopped
1 head broccoli
1 vegetable stock cube made into 300 ml with boiling water

Heat the oil, cooking the garlic and onion until soft. Add a teaspoon of finely chopped coriander, turmeric and chillies. Stir and cook for 2 minutes. Add carrots, sweet potato or squash and tomatoes. Add the liquid stock and chick peas, bring to the boil and then simmer for approximately 20 minutes. Meanwhile, blanch the broccoli and add once the curry is cooked. Remove from the heat; allow to cool slightly before adding the yoghurt. Sprinkle a generous helping of fresh coriander on top and serve with brown rice.

Kedgeree

Ingredients for 2 people

100 g brown rice
2 haddock or mackerel fillets
2 organic eggs
1 tsp turmeric

Cook the rice as usual. Meanwhile poach the fish in water or skimmed milk. Mix the cooked brown rice with the fish and add 1 teaspoon of turmeric. Chop the boiled egg on top and add some fresh coriander or dill.

Tomato soup

Ingredients for 2 people

1 tbs olive oil
8 medium tomatoes, chopped
1 red chilli, de-seeded and chopped
1 onion, grated
2 garlic cloves, crushed
Half a pint vegetable stock
2 tbs chopped parsley, coriander or basil

Heat the oil and cook the onion and chilli. Add the garlic and heat for another 2 minutes. Add the chopped tomatoes and cook for 10 minutes. Add the stock, bring to the boil and then simmer for 20 minutes. Alternatively, this can be cooked in a slow cooker on low for 5–6 hours. Puree the soup in a blender and serve, adding the freshly chopped parsley or basil.

Savoy cabbage stir fry

Ingredients for 2 people

1 onion
2 cloves garlic
1 cup mixed peppers, sweetcorn and peas
2 cups shredded Savoy cabbage
1 tbs mixed seeds or pine nuts
1 red chilli, de-seeded and chopped
Olive oil
Optional extra – organic soya

Chop the garlic, cabbage and onions and add to a teaspoon of heated olive oil in a pan. Once browned, add seeds and vegetables, cook through and serve!

Salmon, sweet potato and rocket risotto

Ingredients for 1 person

1 salmon steak
1 small onion, sliced
2 cloves garlic, thinly sliced
75 g organic brown rice
2 large handfuls rocket
Olive oil
1 medium sweet potato/squash/carrots, roasted

Bake a salmon steak and roast a combination of squash, carrots or sweet potato. Meanwhile, cook the risotto as follows: sauté some garlic and onion with a little olive oil. Add the rice, stirring to coat it with the oil/onion/garlic mixture, then add water and allow to simmer (instructions on rice packets will state how much rice per serving and how much water to use). Keep adding water as required until the rice is cooked. Once all the water is absorbed, add the roasted vegetables and baked salmon to the risotto and serve. Spinach or rocket can also be stirred into the risotto just before serving.

Seared tuna steak

Ingredients for 1 person

1 tuna steak
1 small onion, sliced
2 cloves garlic, thinly sliced
1 portion broccoli
1 medium sweet potato
Olive oil

Heat a little olive oil in a pan and then add the tuna steak. Sear on one side and then turn over and add the onions and garlic. Serve with baked sweet potato or squash, and steamed broccoli. This can also be eaten with garlic roast squash, carrot and sweet potatoes and cruciferous or leafy vegetables such as broccoli or spinach, or with a portion of stir fried vegetables.

Chilli bean stew

Ingredients for 2 people

Selection of beans/lentils, soaked
1 onion, chopped
2 cloves garlic, chopped
1–2 chillis, chopped
2 tsp turmeric
75 g organic brown rice per person
1 cup fresh tomatoes
Olive oil
1 vegetable stock cube made into 300 ml with boiling water

Soak the beans overnight. Whilst boiling the beans, brown the garlic and onion in a little olive oil then add the chillies and turmeric. Add the beans to the dish with the vegetable stock. Simmer for 1 hour or as required. Fresh or tinned tomatoes may be added if desired, along with any other vegetables, lentils and other pulses not requiring pre-soaking. Serve with brown rice.

Stuffed baked vegetables

Ingredients for 2 people

2 large peppers, raw, with tops cut off
2 sweet potatoes still in skins
1 onion, chopped
2 cloves garlic, chopped
100 g fresh spinach
Handful fresh or frozen sweetcorn and peas
1 tsp mixed seeds
1 tsp olive oil

Bake the potatoes until cooked. Heat the oil and lightly brown the garlic and onion. Add the peas and sweetcorn and heat through, adding the spinach and seeds. Stir until wilted and remove from the heat. Cut off the top of the sweet potatoes and mash with the stir-fry mixture, keeping the skin intact. Once thoroughly mixed, stuff the peppers and sweet potatoes with the mixture of stir-fried vegetables, mash and mixed seeds, and bake for 25 minutes at to 180°C/gas mark 4. Serve with a large green salad or broccoli florets.

Salmon and stir fry vegetables

Ingredients for 2 people

2 salmon steaks
2 cloves garlic, sliced
1 small onion, sliced
1 cup mixed peppers
1 cupful of sweetcorn and peas
1 cup shredded Savoy cabbage or spinach
Olive oil

Bake a salmon steak. Meanwhile, heat a little olive oil and add onions, garlic, peppers, sweetcorn, peas, etc. Cook through – this can be mixed with cooked brown rice or rice noodles or served separately.

_____

Getting the most from superfoods

MAXIMUM NUTRITION

Although all of these foods have earned superfood status, the truth is that they are only superfoods if the nutrients are still present and active in the food. There are many farming, storage, food preparation and cooking practices that drastically reduce the nutrient content of our food, so if you really want to feel the benefits of what a superfood diet can do for you, maximize the nutrient content by following as many of these tips as possible:

▶ *Buy or grow organic fruit and vegetables.*
▶ *Use organic, fresh raw garlic in dishes wherever possible.*
▶ *Organize an organic box to be delivered from your local farm scheme.*
▶ *Use free range eggs, unfarmed fish and organically reared meat.*
▶ *Use foods that are not genetically modified (for example, non-GM soya).*
▶ *Eat fresh fruit and vegetables that have been grown locally so that you know how long it has been since the food was harvested.*
▶ *Try to eat fresh food soon after you have bought it.*
▶ *Avoid chopping fruit and vegetables up into small pieces, as the more the food is exposed to the air and light, the higher the loss of anti-oxidant nutrients such as beta carotene and vitamin C.*
▶ *Try to eat plenty of raw fruit and vegetables to maximize nutrient content. An exception here is the tomato, as more of the carotenoid lycopene becomes available once the tomato has been cooked.*

Having said all of this, with a busy lifestyle or tight budget, it may be difficult to do many of these things. If you can't afford organic food and only have time for one food shop weekly from the local supermarket, you can still maximize your nutrient content with the following tips.

SUPERFOODS ON A BUDGET

▶ *Find a local farm that sells organic produce – it may well be less expensive than supermarket prices, especially if you pick it up yourself.*
▶ *Grow your own fruit, vegetables or herbs for really fresh produce and to cut down on the food shopping bill.*
▶ *See if any neighbours or friends have fruit trees, herb gardens, vegetable patches or free range chickens and would consider supplying you.*

SUPERFOODS WITH NO SPARE TIME

▶ *Cut vegetables in bigger chunks – this reduces meal preparation time in itself!*
▶ *Use tinned tomatoes in recipes.*
▶ *Eat a piece of fruit rather than fruit salads – save the time spent preparing a fruit salad, and enjoy a higher nutrient content at the same time!*
▶ *Buy ready-washed salad leaves but try to avoid using pre-chopped, prepared salads too regularly as the nutrient content is drastically reduced in these.*
▶ *Use fresh soups in cartons (not packet or tinned soups), and add a handful of fresh herbs to increase the nutrient content.*

THINGS TO REMEMBER

You can see how easy it is to follow a superfood diet – just follow these simple guidelines:

- *Make every meal a naturally colourful meal.*

- *Choose darker green salad leaves for maximum nutrient content.*

- *Eat raw or lightly cooked vegetables unless stated otherwise (e.g. tomatoes, squash).*

- *Eat garlic and onion daily.*

- *Eat organic and fresh, unprocessed foods for higher nutrient content.*

- *Consume foods such as oats, soy and fish for their special therapeutic properties.*

- *Don't forget beverages, herbs and spices can be superfoods too! (Think green tea and turmeric!)*

Superfood challenge

Try to include at least one of the following in every meal or snack, aiming for one of each at lunch and dinner:

- *green leafy or cruciferous vegetable*

- *onion or garlic*

- *red/orange fruit or vegetable*

- *purple fruit, juice or salad vegetable.*

4

How to detox!

In this chapter you will learn:
* *whether you need to detox*
* *how to detox*
* *about different levels of detox.*

A detox diet is usually undertaken to eliminate toxins from the body, although it has several other benefits and often also results in weight loss through the reduced calorie intake. Although some weight loss is usual during such a regime, detoxification should be done for health, not weight loss, although a healthy detox diet such as the one in this chapter can be a motivating way to kick start a weight-loss programme and less restrictive levels of the detox can be followed for longer periods of time, contributing to healthy weight maintenance.

Get started straight away with a simple daily detox!

▶ *Start each day with a drink of hot water – you can add a slice of lime or lemon for added refreshment.*
▶ *Drink 2 litres of water throughout the day.*
▶ *Eat garlic and onions daily.*
▶ *Eat at least one green leafy vegetable daily.*

The idea of a detoxification diet is to give the liver, digestion and immune system the opportunity to eliminate toxins and boost overall health. Whilst this is a normal process that occurs continuously, if we consume large amounts of products that require detoxification, such as alcohol, caffeine and artificial food additives, for example, it follows that our body may become overloaded and become less effective. Equally, we require certain nutrients for our detoxification systems to work, and a poor diet may leave us unable to detoxify everything that we consume successfully.

The products that we generally eat and drink have been certified as being safe to consume and are not immediately 'toxic' to us, though it could easily be argued that any alcohol consumption has toxic effects within the body. However, there are many compounds that the body has to convert into a toxin before elimination and it is these toxins, which are by-products of the first stage of detoxification, that can damage our health, along with several by-products of normal metabolism. Naturopathic medicine links a number of disease conditions to dysfunctional, overloaded detoxification processes.

Why detox?

Detoxing is done to give the whole body a rest from the daily intake of refined, processed foods and anti-nutrients such as tobacco, caffeine and alcohol that we consume. You may benefit from a detoxification diet if you smoke, consume large amounts of alcohol and/or caffeine daily, or if you eat a nutrient-poor diet that consists of mostly packaged, convenience foods. This type of lifestyle is likely to result in symptoms and health conditions that would indicate the need for a detox – check out the following list to see if you might benefit! Tick the symptoms that apply to you – this will help you to decide not only whether you need to detox, but also what level of detox to choose later on in this chapter.

Fatigue and poor energy levels ☐

Regular headaches ☐

Cloudy urine ☐

Irregular bowel function ☐

Constipation ☐

Haemorrhoids ☐

Yellowed sclera (whites of the eyes) ☐

Elevated cholesterol levels ☐

Gallstones or kidney stones ☐

Digestive disorders ☐

Food allergies ☐

Poor quality sleep or insomnia ☐

Menstrual problems ☐

Thrush or other yeast infection
(for example, athlete's foot) ☐

Skin problems, spots and rashes ☐

Although these are key symptoms indicating sluggish liver and bowel function, there are many others that could be added. The list is so diverse because the liver is our main organ of detoxification and if it is overloaded, because of its many essential roles in the body, it affects many different body systems. One of the first systems that liver dysfunction affects is that of the bowel as these two organs are directly linked, so if one is under-functioning, it affects the other.

DETOX BENEFITS

With so many body systems affected by sub-optimal liver function, it follows that the list of benefits a detox can offer is also quite diverse. Detox benefits can include any or all of the following:

- ▶ *weight loss*
- ▶ *glowing skin and hair*
- ▶ *reduction in cellulite and fatty tissue*
- ▶ *reduced abdominal bloating and water retention*
- ▶ *better digestive function*

- *improved bowel function*
- *improved energy levels*
- *improved mental clarity and mood*
- *enhanced immune function*
- *improved quality of sleep.*

A detox regime can run over a day or over months, and can range from being a stringent fruit and water-only regime to a healthy diet that is a way of life, enabling ongoing detoxification as nature intended it. With any type of dietary adjustment lasting more than a couple of days, it is important that you take advice from a dietician or nutritionist and first check out your health with your doctor.

Do YOU need to detox?

Many experts state that as detoxification is an ongoing, natural process, there is no need for a specific detox. However, it is also true that some of us consume higher levels of toxins, or may not have effective systems of detoxification. Even if you have none of the symptoms listed opposite, all of the things listed below increase your likelihood of benefiting from a detox:

- *smoking or passive smoking*
- *high alcohol intake (above the recommended levels of 14 units per week for women, or 21 units for men, although some individuals may have a lower threshold)*
- *high intake of processed foods containing additives*
- *low intake of anti-oxidants such as vitamin A, carotenes, Vitamin C, Vitamin E, zinc and selenium*
- *low intake of the foods that aid detoxification (proteins, garlic, onions, broccoli, etc.)*
- *Low water intake*
- *Low fibre intake.*

If you answered 'yes' to three or more statements, a change in diet and lifestyle is recommended and you will probably benefit from some type of detox. However, detox isn't necessarily the name of the diet you will follow – it is the word describing what your body will naturally do given the opportunity, with enough energy and an ample supply of nutrients. All you need to do is two things:

1 *Lighten the load by eating a healthier diet (reducing intake of products that require detoxification).*
2 *Increase your intake of the nutrients your body needs to help with detoxification.*

However, if you eat healthily for the majority of the time, you can enjoy the same benefits that a detoxification diet would bring, without any major adjustments to your lifestyle and diet! The lower toxin intake and higher nutrient content in a healthy diet allows your body to detoxify as required on an ongoing basis, reducing the need for a specific detox diet.

Let's take a quick look at what toxins are and how the detox process works before deciding on the level of detox to suit you. If, however, you want to get started straight away, you can skip forwards to 'Detox options'.

What are toxins?

Toxins are substances that have no use in the body, and may cause damage if left circulating or stored within our cells.

▶ **Endotoxins** *are products left at the end of metabolic reactions in the body.*
▶ **Exotoxins** *are substances taken in, such as drugs, chemicals, pollutants, etc.*

Some toxins, particularly fat-soluble toxins, are stored in adipose tissue (fat) and these become mobilized within the body whenever we lose body fat. As fat is used up for energy, it releases the contents of its cells, including any toxins. These enter the circulation and can make us feel nauseous or ill – trade-mark symptoms of many detox diets.

Regularly consumed substances that require detoxification in the liver:

- *coffee*
- *cooked meats*
- *other 'charcoaled' products*
- *some food additives*
- *products from cigarette smoke*
- *alcohol.*

How we detoxify

Detoxification is mostly done in the liver, with some detoxification taking place in the intestines. The liver filters and detoxifies products which may be harmful, although some substances are turned into more harmful substances before they are eliminated from the body, which is why detoxification must be followed by successful elimination. The detoxification process happens in three phases.

Nutrients needed for Phase 1 detoxification in the liver

Amino acids including glutathione (from protein)
*Flavonoids (for example, quercetin from onions)
Vitamins B_2, B_3, B_{12}
Phospholipids (from eggs, soya beans)
*See Chapter 3 for a list of flavonoid-rich foods.

PHASE 1 OF DETOXIFICATION

▶ *Toxins undergo a chemical reaction with enzymes in the liver.*

We need several nutrients for Phase 1 detoxification.

Part of the detoxification process includes quenching destructive free radicals. Free radicals are molecules or atoms which are unstable – see Chapter 6 for more information on free radical damage. Free radicals can be stabilized or 'disarmed' from being destructive by anti-oxidants, which 'quench' free radicals. Anti-oxidants can be found throughout the tissues in the body and are an important part of the detoxification process.

Anti-oxidants and the foods that contain them:

▶ *carotenes (found in carrots, sweet potato, squash, apricots, etc.)*
▶ *bioflavonoids (often found in citrus fruits)*
▶ *vitamin C (found in peppers, citrus fruits, berries, green leafy vegetables)*
▶ *vitamin E (found in nuts, seeds, avocados, vegetable oils)*
▶ *zinc (found in whole grains, seafood, meats, pumpkin seeds)*
▶ *selenium (found in Brazil nuts, sunflower seeds, brown rice, seafood)*
▶ *copper (found in mushrooms, offal and seafood)*
▶ *manganese (found mostly in leafy vegetables and seafood)*
▶ *co-enzyme Q10 (synthesized in tissues but also found in offal, beef, soya)*
▶ *anti-oxidant compounds found in garlic, onions and cruciferous vegetables (for example, broccoli).*

PHASE 2 OF DETOXIFICATION

▶ *A water-soluble compound is then added to the toxin to help remove it from the body.*
▶ *Many water-soluble compounds are amino acids, found in protein foods such as fish, soya, eggs or meat, as well as in plant foods.*

- *Vitamin A and foods such as garlic and onions are also essential for some Phase 2 reactions.*
- *Toxins that have been made water soluble are excreted via the kidneys.*
- *Fat-soluble (and some water-soluble) toxins are excreted in the faeces.*

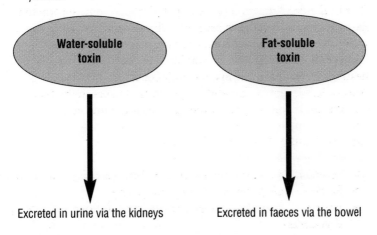

Figure 4.1 *Phase 2 of detoxification.*

> It is important that Phase 2 of detoxification can cope with the toxic substances produced in Phase 1. Substances such as cigarette smoke or alcohol increase the first phase of detoxification, and if these new toxins are not further metabolized in Phase 2, they can react with our DNA and protein molecules in our cells, causing cellular damage.

Elimination

This is an essential part of the detoxification process, and is often overlooked. There is little point 'detoxifying' and moving toxins from our cells into our circulation, if we then fail to eliminate these products from the body. Extra toxins circulating in the bloodstream is one of the reasons for the side effects often experienced during a detox, such as feeling nauseous – if we don't eliminate the toxins from our body, they simply circulate for a while and then return to our cells, meaning that your detox has been a waste of time.

Organs of elimination:

- *the bowel (and colon)*
- *the kidneys*
- *the skin*
- *the lungs.*

The two organs that should ideally be eliminating toxins are the bowel and kidneys. If the body is overloaded with toxins, or elimination is not effective enough, toxins can be eliminated via the lungs or skin, causing excess mucus or spots.

You can enhance your toxin elimination by maximizing kidney and bowel function as follows:

1 *Drink plenty of water.*
2 *Eat plenty of high-fibre foods such as brown rice.*

Water provides a vehicle by which toxins can be eliminated via the kidneys and it also ensures good bowel motility, reducing the risk of constipation. In the digestive tract, fibre absorbs both water-soluble and fat-soluble toxins and removes toxins via the faeces. Brown rice is often used by naturopaths as it is a very effective source of fibre, capable of absorbing and eliminating by-products of detoxification, excess cholesterol and drugs.

If you cannot consume brown rice for any reason, other complex carbohydrates such as corn, millet flakes, quinoa, porridge oats or potatoes can be substituted.

Detox options

So, now you need to decide on the level of detox to suit you – a detox can vary in intensity and duration. Look at these options and considerations to help you decide on your detox plan.

Detox options

Quick but intense	A detox consuming nothing but water, fruit and vegetables for two days.
Takes more time but easier to do	A healthy eating plan which allows the body to detoxify gradually over a number of weeks.
Mix and match	Eat a generally healthy diet for most of the time, but have more stringent detox days every couple of weeks.

Other options ...

▶ *You can adjust the level of detox to suit your lifestyle, fitting around work, social and family occasions.*
▶ *You can dip in and out of the different levels in this detox plan.*

Insight: Detox tip

Detox will work better if it is done over a longer period of time – at least three to four days – and if you move from one level to another in stages. This gives your body longer to adjust to dietary changes, and extends the length of time with allergens and heavy protein foods excluded from the diet, which in turn provides more opportunity for detoxification.

DIFFERENT LEVELS OF DETOX

Level 1 Omit confectionary, tea, coffee, alcohol, packet and tinned food and refined carbohydrates – cut out all the rubbish!

Level 2 Eliminate meat, eggs, dairy produce and wheat from the diet.

Level 3 Remove fish and soya products and other grains except rice.

Level 4   You may spend a day on just fruit, vegetables, water and juices, having eliminated brown rice, nuts and seeds.

So, you need to decide how long you would like to spend on the detox and how stringent you would like it to be. Whatever you decide, you should not spend more than a day at Level 3 or Level 4 as these levels are excluding important food groups such as proteins, starchy carbohydrates and fatty acids which are required for good health.

Levels 1 and 2 – long-stay options

If you would like to extend your detox over a longer period of time, this will give your body more opportunity to detoxify and will also help to create healthier eating habits. You could stay at Level 1 indefinitely, avoiding the products that create the need for a detox in the first place. Living at Level 1 would reduce or even remove the need to follow a specific detox diet again.

Level 2 is also a relatively healthy option to remain at for a while, although if you are pregnant, breastfeeding or have any medical condition you should check with your doctor and consult with a qualified practitioner before you make any radical changes to your diet. For short-term dietary adjustments you can ensure ample calcium intake from nuts and seeds, green leafy vegetables, tinned fish and dried apricots, and obtain iron from dark green leafy vegetables, beans and pulses.

Omitting meat, eggs and dairy foods is similar to a vegan diet but with fish still included – excluding these foods results in a large decrease in saturated fat and cholesterol intake, and will benefit your health and reduce body weight. Protein and essential fatty acids are still included in the form of fish, which has been linked with a lower incidence of heart disease, reduced blood pressure and lower cholesterol levels.

Insight: Cutting out the allergens

Dairy foods, eggs and wheat are the most common foods that people are allergic/sensitive to, so you may find that avoiding these foods alleviates symptoms such as digestive problems, headaches or fatigue. For long-term healthy diets, you may want to try re-introducing eggs and exclude meat, wheat or dairy, or eat these foods sparingly. Some people with food sensitivity re-introduce foods into their diet after a period of exclusion without any adverse reaction, but symptoms may recur if the allergen is eaten too often.

Although it can be difficult on a practical level to avoid wheat as it is so commonly eaten, other carbohydrates such as oats, rice, quinoa or barley easily replace the nutrients normally found in wheat, and so excluding this from the diet is not a problem as long as you replace wheat products with other starchy carbohydrates. It can be difficult to avoid wheat when you are not at home or preparing your own meals, as so many commercial products contain wheat – sandwiches, pasta, cereals, biscuits, pastries, etc. Wheat is also often used as a cheap filler in many processed food products.

Levels 3 and 4 – short stay only

Level 3 is not a healthy long-term eating plan – it simply removes the remaining protein foods (fish and soya products) and grains other than rice to give the digestive system, liver and immune system a 'rest' and opportunity to offload and eliminate toxins. Nuts and seeds may still be included at this point. We require protein, fatty acids and starchy carbohydrates for health, so these foods should not be omitted long term. The remaining fruit, vegetables, juices, nuts, seeds, rice and water provide many of the nutrients required for detoxification, and the rice and water aid elimination. You should not remain at Level 3 for longer than a day.

After a day at Level 3 you may begin to 'reverse' the detox, bringing foods back into the diet in the reverse order that they were eliminated, or you may choose to spend one day at Level 4, consuming just fruit, vegetables, juices and water. You may also include some brown rice to aid elimination.

Reversing the detox

After a day at Level 4, you return to spend a day at Level 3 including rice, nuts and seeds in the diet, or may go back to Level 2. This re-introduces some of the foods that are more difficult to digest slowly into the diet, and also prolongs the healthy detox phase by not re-introducing heavy protein foods and common allergens until the last phase.

So now you understand the principle of moving through the different levels of detox, it's time to decide how long you want to spend on the detox plan.

> ### Insight: Option to stay and avoid 're-toxing'
> If you enjoy the way this new way of eating makes you feel and look, why not stay at Level 2 or Level 1 after your detox? Choosing not to re-introduce processed foods, tea, coffee and alcohol into your diet, or maybe avoiding or limiting wheat, meat or dairy foods, will provide you with a healthy eating plan that reduces the need for radical detoxification in the future.

Planning your detox

If you're planning just a day or two of detoxification, you will benefit more from cutting out all the products and foods omitted in Levels 1 and 2, omitting meat, wheat, eggs and dairy as well as all processed foods.

Detox plan A

Friday	Saturday	Sunday
Level 1	Level 2	Level 1

Alternatively, over the same amount of time you could follow a more intense detox by going to Level 3 as shown opposite.

Detox plan B

Friday	Saturday	Sunday
Level 2	Level 3	Level 2

If you have five days or more, simply adapt the number of days at each level to suit the time you have available. For example, a five-day detox might look like this:

Detox plan C

Day 1	Day 2	Day 3	Day 4	Day 5
Level 1	Level 2	Level 3	Level 2	Level 1

A week-long detox will extend the time you spend at one or more levels:

Detox plan D

Day 1	Day 2	Day 3	Day 4	Day 5	Day 6	Day 7
Level 1	Level 2	Level 2	Level 3	Level 4	Level 3	Level 2

Alternatively you could follow the detox plan in this chapter which provides a planned detox over 14 days.

TIMING YOUR DETOX

When planning your detox, make sure you take these things into consideration:

▶ *You may not have the energy to exercise or be overly active.*
▶ *If you are at work or have social engagements over the duration of your detox, you may find it more difficult to eat the foods outlined in the eating plans, and it may be worth planning your detox at another time.*

- ▶ *You should avoid driving or using any machinery, as your glucose levels may be lower than usual, and this affects mental clarity and concentration.*
- ▶ *You should plan a day of total relaxation, maybe a massage or a long bath to coincide with the peak of your detox, especially if you plan to spend a day at Level 4.*

SHOPPING LIST

Once you have decided on the level of detox to suit you, you will need to buy the foods and drinks you need to follow the detox plan. As with any eating plan, the first step towards success is in the planning and preparation – if you haven't got the foods you need at home for your detox, it will be short lived! This is a list of items that are included in the detox eating plan – you will need to decide on the amounts you will need depending upon how long your detox will be for:

- ✓ *Apples, lemons, limes, oranges, grapefruit, red grapes, mangoes, papayas, apricots, a selection of berries, kiwi, bananas plus any other fresh fruit of your choice.*
- ✓ *A selection of green salad leaves including chicory, spinach, watercress and rocket, beetroot, tomatoes, cucumber, celery, radishes, onions, red onions, asparagus, garlic, avocado, whole peppers, mushrooms.*
- ✓ *Sweet potatoes, squash, broccoli, cauliflower, Brussels sprouts, Savoy or spring cabbage, peas, sweetcorn, carrots, parsnips.*
- ✓ *Ingredients to make soup at home, or fresh soup in cartons (look for low-salt, low-fat vegetable options: tomato, asparagus, mixed vegetable, lentil soups) and hummus if not making home-made hummus (chick peas, olive oil and garlic).*
- ✓ *Brown rice, chickpeas, lentils, beans and pulses (ideally ready to soak, but tinned can be used), quinoa, barley (for home-made soups), rice cakes or corn cakes.*
- ✓ *Milk (soya, oat or rice), live yoghurt, free range organic eggs, a variety of fish, lean meats and skimmed milk for the beginning and end of the detox if desired, unsalted nuts and seeds, nut/seed bars and olive oil.*

✓ *Porridge oats, muesli or another cereal for the beginning and end of the detox if desired.*

✓ *Bottled water if necessary, herbal teas, green tea, coffee alternatives such as dandelion coffee or Barley Cup (optional), turmeric, chillies, fresh herbs (coriander, parsley, basil, dill, etc.).*

Top ten foods for detox

Amongst this shopping list are several foods/food groups which will really contribute to an effective detox – these foods should ideally be eaten regularly in your usual diet, but should be included daily during a detox:

▶ *onions*
▶ *garlic*
▶ *green leafy vegetables (spinach, watercress, rocket)*
▶ *cruciferous vegetables (broccoli, sprouts, cabbage, cauliflower)*
▶ *a range of beta carotene-rich foods (sweet potatoes, mango, carrots)*
▶ *a range of vitamin C-rich foods (peppers, kiwi, berries, citrus fruit)*
▶ *water (though not a food, it is a truly essential element in this diet)*
▶ *avocado for vitamin E and fatty acids*
▶ *Brazil nuts for selenium, fatty acids and vitamin E*
▶ *seeds for bowel motility, essential fatty acids, mineral and vitamins.*

Other things to help:

▶ *a steamer for vegetables*
▶ *a juicer for juicing fresh fruits*
▶ *a blender for smoothies*
▶ *body brushing helps to stimulate movement within the lymph system from where fat and toxins are released, carrying them*

to the bloodstream and the kidneys or bowel for elimination. Body brushing or massage (lymphatic or otherwise) enhances circulation and aids toxin elimination, so if you have a body brush, make use of it! You should brush towards the lymph nodes in the groin and the armpits.

▶ Epsom salts baths are also often recommended during a detox as the salts (magnesium sulphate) are said to increase perspiration and help draw toxins out of the skin.

Basic detox guidelines

Important points to remember are:

▶ Make sure you drink lots of water – up to 2 litres daily.
▶ Start each day with a mug or glass of hot water. For an extra detox boost, add a squeeze and slice of fresh lemon or lime, or add a little unsweetened red grape or apple juice to your hot water. You can drink this throughout the day if you prefer it to cold water.
▶ Make sure that you eat enough to maintain energy levels and sustain normal blood glucose levels – if you feel lethargic, dizzy or faint, you aren't eating enough!
▶ Remove foods from your diet gradually, and re-introduce eliminated foods back into the diet gradually, in reverse order to that in which they were originally taken out.

HOW WATER HELPS DURING A DETOX

1 It keeps faeces in the bowel well lubricated, aiding in its removal from the body.
2 Water-soluble toxins and end products can be removed from the body via the kidneys in urine, and water helps this process.

During a detox you should aim to drink more than normal, although some of this can come from the foods that you eat such as melons, cucumber or tomatoes which all have a high water content.

HERBAL TEAS AND OTHER ALTERNATIVES

One of the most difficult elements of following a detox regime can be giving up tea and coffee. Due to the physiological effect of the caffeine in these drinks, you can easily experience 'withdrawal' symptoms such as a headache or moodiness if you are used to a regular caffeine fix. De-caffeinated drinks aren't a realistic option during a detox as these contain several chemical residues that are left in the product after the caffeine has been removed, and some caffeine often still remains. The best way to reduce your intake of all caffeinated drinks, including carbonated drinks such as cola, is to do it gradually to allow your body a period of adjustment to the change. You can do this by:

▶ *reducing the number of drinks you have each day*
▶ *using a smaller cup instead of a large mug*
▶ *making your tea or coffee weaker than usual.*

It is essential that you have alternative drinks to replace your usual beverage, and there are many different types of herbal tea and other healthier alternatives to try. Good alternatives for coffee drinkers include products such as Barley Cup or Dandelion coffee. If you want alternative options to a mug of hot water with a slice of lemon or lime, or splash of red grape or apple juice, there are hundreds of herbal teas available, with many of them offering medicinal properties which can contribute to your detox. Here are just a few suggestions:

Peppermint tea or chamomile tea	Calming, aiding relaxation and sleep. Can aid digestion especially if heartburn or irritable bowel syndrome is present.

(Contd)

Ginger tea	Can also aid digestion, improve circulation and may reduce headaches.
Lemon tea or nettle tea	Support liver function.

Insight: Other healthy tea alternatives

Green tea and Rooibosch (red bush) tea are more similar to normal tea. Rooibosch tea is caffeine-free and has a lower tannin content than normal tea. Green tea contains much less caffeine than a normal cup of tea or coffee, and possesses several health benefits including anti-oxidants which support immune function. More information on the anti-oxidant catechins in green tea can be found in Chapter 3.

Supplements to help

A detox diet is likely to be very different from your normal dietary regime and as such, this should produce significant results in your health and possibly in your body weight. Supplements can help to support a successful detox regime by either improving elimination of toxins from the body, easing symptoms experienced during detoxification, providing essential nutrients needed for detoxification, or boosting liver function. Although none of these supplements are essential, you may find some of them helpful.

MILK THISTLE (SILYMARIN)

This herb stimulates liver function and as such aids the detoxification process. Milk thistle is available in several formats including capsules and homeopathic drops.

LECITHIN (PHOSPHATIDYL CHOLINE)

This nutrient supports liver function and works very well in conjunction with Silymarin (milk thistle). Research has shown that taking it alongside milk thistle can increase the effectiveness of the Silymarin herb.

MULTI-VITAMIN, MULTI-MINERAL CAPSULES OR ANTI-OXIDANTS

Without the expert advice of a dietician or registered nutritionist, you should opt for a supplement that offers a wide range of vitamins and minerals in one capsule. This is because several of these micronutrients work together, and occur together naturally in foods. If taken in isolation, some nutrients can create imbalances in the body, so this should only be done if advised by a qualified practitioner. Watch out for the nutrients needed for detoxification:

- *beta carotene*
- *vitamin C*
- *vitamin E*
- *zinc*
- *selenium*
- *manganese*
- *copper*
- *B vitamins.*

You will get the amino acids you need from protein foods, the other compounds such as flavonoids are included in the detox diet. Nutrient supplements should be taken with food; if you are pregnant, breastfeeding or taking any medication, you should check with your doctor first.

PSYLLIUM HUSK POWDER

This is a natural fibre that is added to water or juice. It aids bowel motility and can be used to increase bowel elimination or if constipation or diarrhoea are experienced during the detox. It is essential to consume plenty of fluid if you take psyllium husks to ensure that the extra fibre eases constipation instead of contributing to it – we need to drink extra water whenever we take in additional fibre.

Case study

Marcus had irritable bowel syndrome and suffered with both chronic diarrhoea and constipation. Within one week of using psyllium husk fibre, his bowel movements had become regular and easy, bulking out the stool to avoid diarrhoea, and aiding peristalsis, which reduced the constipation.

What to expect during your detox

Whenever you lower your food intake, you should be prepared for reduced blood sugar levels which may make you feel lethargic, 'fuzzy headed' or even a little dizzy, although you should aim to avoid this by eating regularly throughout the day and making sure that you eat enough. It is recommended that you take plenty of rest during a detox, especially with more stringent dietary regimes.

If your usual diet is high in toxins, just changing to a healthy eating regime may initially make you feel worse. For example:

▶ *When you first begin to drink lots of water, you may be visiting the toilet more regularly, but as your body becomes accustomed to the new hydration levels this will settle down.*
▶ *Giving up caffeine can be difficult. If you've tried to cut out tea or coffee before, you may have suffered with a headache that just wouldn't budge without your daily fix. Try to reduce your caffeine intake slowly and use healthier alternatives such as green tea or Barley Cup.*

Many people suffer with flatulence when they increase their intake of fibre, but it's really worth giving your body (and bowels) time to adjust as a high-fibre diet provides several health benefits. The main flatulence-causing culprits are foods from the bean and pulse family; however, these foods are an excellent source of fibre, starch, vegetable protein, minerals and vitamins, so it's worth trying to incorporate some beans into your diet.

If you're giving up lots of sugary or refined foods (sweets, chocolate, white bread, biscuits etc.), you might find yourself feeling lethargic and craving sugars. Keep your blood sugar levels constant with lots of slow-release carbohydrates such as porridge, pulses and green vegetables, eaten together with proteins such as fish and soya.

Insight

Chew your food thoroughly to avoid taking in too much air with food, and make sure you eat a combination of fruit, vegetables, beans and oats (high in soluble fibre) as well as foods such as wholegrain bread, which contains more insoluble fibre.

Possible side effects

The end products of detoxification have to be eliminated from the body via the bowel and the kidneys, and may also be eliminated via the skin and lungs. If any of these organs are functioning below par, or if the level of toxins to be eliminated is very high, symptoms such as headaches, constipation, spots, a cough or a cold may be experienced. You can ease these symptoms by either:

▶ *'cutting back' on the strength of the detox, by returning to a less restrictive level, i.e. re-introducing some foods previously omitted; or*
▶ *increasing elimination by drinking more water (to aid elimination through the kidneys) and eating more brown rice (aiding elimination through the bowel).*

As drugs such as headache tablets have to undergo detoxification in the liver, it is recommended that you try to avoid these, and ease any symptoms naturally through adjusting your diet as above, relaxation, sleep or a relaxing treatment such as a massage.

As toxins move from the cells to be eliminated from the body, this increase in toxicity may cause the following symptoms, particularly if you can't eliminate them quickly enough. You can either ease back on the strength of the detox (though if you ease all the way back to your normal diet your detox is effectively ended!), or aim to ease your symptoms through naturopathic means as follows.

A COUGH, COLD OR EXCESS MUCUS PRODUCTION

Increase elimination through the kidneys and bowel by drinking more water and eating more rice, fruit and vegetables. This will take pressure off the respiratory system as toxins are removed through the normal channels. Try to avoid taking any medication for your cold or cough as this will simply add to your toxic load.

CYSTITIS

Drink plenty of fluids and include cranberry juice, cranberries or blueberries in your diet. Cranberries and blueberries contain proanthocyanidins which can make bacterial adherence to the lining of the bladder or urethra more difficult, reducing infection and aiding recovery. (See Chapter 3 for more information on these plant nutrients.)

DIARRHOEA OR CONSTIPATION

Increase your intake of brown rice as the fibre can help bulk up the stool (and help reduce diarrhoea) or aid bowel motility (reducing constipation). Stewed fruit will help with constipation due to the high content of water and soluble fibre. A useful supplement is a natural fibre called psyllium husk which can be bought from health food shops. Adding a teaspoon of this fibre to juice or water each day will help to prevent constipation and can also bulk out the stool. If you suffer with either diarrhoea or constipation, you must increase your water intake to replace lost fluids and aid bowel movement.

SPOTS, RASHES OR CYSTS

Try not to use any medications or skin lotions during your detox as these simply block any elimination through the skin and increase the amount of toxins in the circulation. Keep the skin clean and try not to apply make up or skin care products. A hot bath or steam facial will help to open the pores and enhance elimination – remember these are all symptoms of elimination which should be encouraged rather than blocked. Topical application of diluted Aloe Vera juice (also available from health food shops) may be helpful to reduce inflammation, itching and redness.

HEADACHES

A headache can be a sign of a blocked bowel or poor liver function, and may be alleviated through enhanced bowel motility and detoxification. Try to relax or sleep, drink plenty of water and ensure that bowel movement is regular (at least daily). Use stewed fruit, brown rice, fluids and psyllium husk to improve bowel motility.

However, if a detoxification diet is managed properly, unwelcome side effects should be minimal, if they occur at all. If any health conditions seem severe or continue you should seek advice from your doctor.

The detox plan – elimination and re-introduction of foods

Level	What to cut out and re-introduce	What to eat
Level 1	Eliminate confectionary, tea, coffee, alcohol, packet and tinned food, refined carbohydrates	Fresh meat, eggs and fish, fruit, vegetables, juices, whole grains and dairy foods
Level 2	Eliminate dairy produce, eggs, meat and wheat	Fish, rice, soya products, oats, fruit and vegetables, nuts and seeds

(Contd)

Level 3	Remove fish and soya products, and all grains except brown rice	Brown rice, nuts, seeds, fruits, juices and vegetables
Level 4 (optional)	Eliminate brown rice, nuts and seeds	Fruits, juices and vegetables (1 day only)
Level 3	Re-introduce brown rice, nuts and seeds	Brown rice, vegetables, seeds, fruits and juices
Level 2	Re-introduce fish, soya and other grains apart from wheat. You may choose to remain at this level	Fish, soya products, rice, oats, fruit, nuts, seeds, juices and vegetables
Level 1	Re-introduce meat, eggs, wheat and dairy foods. You may decide to eat only organically reared meat or consume low fat dairy products. You may choose to remain at this level.	Fresh meat or fish, eggs, vegetables, fruit, juices, all whole grains and dairy foods.
Normal eating...	Re-introduce confectionary, alcohol, cigarettes, tea and coffee, refinedcarbohydrates, tinned and packet foods – if you must!	Anything you like! But remember, the more you consume processed, refined foods, alcohol, tea and coffee, the more you'll need to detox again!

Fourteen-day detox eating plan

Day 1/Level 1 (Anti-nutrients and processed foods removed)

Breakfast	1 cup of muesli with soya or rice milk, banana and berries
Mid-morning	Smoothie – 1 cup of blueberries whizzed up with a little milk, a banana and a dessertspoonful of live yoghurt
Lunch	Tomato or vegetable soup
Dinner	Turkey or chicken breast with vegetable stir fry

Day 2/Level 1 (Anti-nutrients and processed foods removed)

Breakfast	Live yoghurt drizzled with honey, served with chopped banana and mixed seeds
Mid-morning	Hummus with raw carrot, celery and peppers
Lunch	Couscous or brown rice salad
Dinner	Seared tuna steak with vegetable stir fry – onion, mushroom, peppers, peas and sweetcorn

Day 3/Level 1 (Anti-nutrients and processed foods removed)

Breakfast	1 cupful of bran flakes or muesli with skimmed/soya milk and mixed berries
Mid-morning	Raw vegetable crudités with low fat yoghurt or hummus dip
Lunch	1 scrambled egg and a cupful of baked beans with 1 slice wholemeal toast
Dinner	Vegetable risotto (add turkey mince or salmon if desired)

Day 4/Level 2 (Meat, dairy, eggs and wheat removed)

Breakfast
Porridge made with water or soya/rice milk, with fruit

Mid-morning
Wheat-free oat or nut/seed bar

Lunch
Grilled sardines with a green salad, tomatoes, onion, beetroot

Dinner
Salmon steak with baked sweet potato, broccoli, cauliflower

Day 5/Level 2 (Meat, dairy, eggs and wheat removed)

Breakfast
Porridge made with water, soya or rice milk. Add a teaspoon of mixed seeds and raspberries

Mid-morning
Smoothie – 1 cup of blueberries whizzed up with some water and soya yoghurt

Lunch
Tomato or vegetable soup

Dinner
Marinated tofu with stir-fried vegetables

Day 6/Level 3 (Fish, soya and most grains removed)

Breakfast
Mixed berries and banana smoothie (berries, banana, water)

Mid-morning
Snack on fruit or fruit salad, rice cakes, nuts and seeds

Lunch
Raw spinach salad with avocado, asparagus, tomatoes, cucumber, red onion and diced beetroot

Dinner
Vegetable and rice-stuffed peppers or aubergine (eggplant)

Day 7/Level 4 (Just fruit, juice and vegetables for a day!)

Breakfast	Fruit salad – mixed berries, banana, grapes, apple and kiwi
Snacks	Fruit and fresh fruit juice throughout the day
Lunch	Home-made tomato, mixed vegetables or lentil soup
Dinner	Vegetable stir fry: onion, garlic, mushroom, peppers, peas, etc.

Day 8/Level 3 (Re-introduce brown rice, nuts and seeds)

Breakfast	Fruit salad – melon, banana, grapes, chopped apple, mango
Snacks	Raw vegetable crudités and fruit
Lunch	Mixed salad leaves, beetroot, tomato, onions, avocado, carrot with rice or corn cakes
Dinner	Vegetable risotto – brown rice mixed with steamed vegetables

Day 9/Level 2 (Re-introduce fish, soya and grains)

Breakfast	Porridge made with water, soya or rice milk. Add a teaspoon of mixed seeds and raspberries
Mid-morning	Hummus with raw carrot and peppers
Lunch	Couscous or brown rice salad
Dinner	Seared tuna steak with vegetable stir fry – onion, mushroom, peppers, peas and corn

Day 10 /Level 2 (No meat, dairy, eggs or wheat for one more day!)

Breakfast	Berries, kiwi, orange/grapefruit segments, banana, grapes with soya yoghurt and mixed seeds
Mid-morning	Rice/corn cakes with mashed banana or avocado
Lunch	Grilled or tinned sardines with a green salad, tomatoes, onions and beetroot
Dinner	Vegetable stew – parsnip, potato, carrot, peas, turnip, swede, parsnip, onion and leek with vegetable gravy or stock

Day 11/Level 1 (Re-introduce dairy, eggs, wheat and meat if desired)

Breakfast	Mixed berry smoothie. Add half a banana, yoghurt or more water to alter thickness as desired
Mid-morning	Cereal or nut/seed bar
Lunch	Mediterranean salad with boiled egg, avocado, steamed asparagus, vine tomatoes, spinach and pine nuts
Dinner	Baked salmon steak with baked sweet potato, broccoli and cauliflower

Day 12/Level 1 (Back to 'normal' diet with healthy eating adjustments!)

Breakfast	Live yoghurt drizzled with honey, served with chopped banana and seeds
Mid-morning	Fruit or fruit salad
Lunch	Chicken salad sandwich on wholemeal bread
Dinner	Vegetable curry and rice

Day 13/Level 1 (Back to 'normal' diet with healthy eating adjustments!)

Breakfast	Porridge made with water, skimmed, soya or rice milk with added fruit and mixed seeds
Snacks	1–2 rice/corn cakes with sliced banana and kiwi
Lunch	Home-made vegetable soup
Dinner	Turkey or chicken breast with peppers, onion, courgette and mushroom kebabs

Day 14/Level 1 (Back to 'normal' diet with healthy eating adjustments!)

Breakfast	Bircher muesli with a dessertspoon of live yoghurt and mixed berries
Mid-morning	Nut/seed or cereal bar
Lunch	Sunday roast – go easy on the meat and potatoes, fill up on vegetables
Dinner	Tuna niscoise salad with a lemon and olive oil dressing

If you decide to return to your original diet and 're-tox' after your detox, you might at least decide to reduce alcohol or caffeine intake, or eat less refined and processed foods. Your body will thank you for it in the long run! Remember, a healthy body isn't just at detox time – it's for life!

THINGS TO REMEMBER

So, for an effective, enjoyable detox experience, don't forget...

- *Plan for success – when is the best time to detox, how long will you detox for, and what foods will you need to shop for?*

- *Drink lots of water.*

- *Detox is not a time to be exerting yourself at work or with exercise – relax!*

- *Gradually eliminate foods from your normal diet, and re-introduce them in reverse order.*

- *Make sure that you eat enough to maintain your energy*

  ... and try not to 're-tox' too much after your detox!

5

Functional foods

In this chapter you will learn:
- *what a functional food is and how it works*
- *whether you need functional foods*
- *what the best functional foods are.*

Functional foods have been around for a long time, previously known as fortified foods – think of breakfast cereals with added vitamins and minerals, or soya with added calcium. You may not be familiar with terms such as functional foods, designer foods or neutraceuticals, but you have almost certainly bought a probiotic drink, a margarine spread which promises to lower cholesterol, or orange juice with added omega 3 oils!

Time-starved but health conscious, we want to get the maximum benefit out of foods with the minimum amount of time and effort expended and functional foods appear to provide this 'quick fix'. By adding ingredients known to enhance health, food manufacturers can make useful nutrients more accessible to us and increase the benefits of buying their product(s) at the same time. So is this a win–win situation?

Although the concept of using foods to either prevent disease or promote health is not new, the functional food market has risen steeply over the last few years. These functional foods are rapidly increasing in popularity, with the 'yoghurt drink' market being one of the fastest growing in the UK and hundreds of new products launched every year. However, you don't have to buy functional foods to enrich your health, although some of them may make it easier for you to improve your diet.

The most well-known functional foods are those with added probiotics, prebiotics, plant sterols and omega 3 fatty acids. Each of these added ingredients offer a different health benefit:

▶ *Prebiotics and probiotics can improve intestinal health.*
▶ *Plant sterols and stanols help to lower cholesterol.*
▶ *Omega 3 fatty acids offer a range of health benefits, but are often added to improve cardiovascular health.*

The market for these functional foods is still increasing, but there is doubt regarding the benefits of many functional foods. As you read through this chapter, you will be able to decide …

1 *whether you need more of the nutrients commonly added to functional foods*
2 *whether buying functional foods is the best way for you to obtain these active ingredients or nutrients.*

In the meantime, you can make your own 'functional foods':

▶ *Add linseeds or linseed oil to yoghurts.*
▶ *Eat fruit with live yoghurt for a prebiotic and probiotic fix.*
▶ *Add chicory, asparagus or garlic to meals to help lower cholesterol.*

What are functional foods?

Functional foods offer extra health benefits in addition to the general nutrition gained from standard foods. Foods may be called functional if they:

1 *naturally contain specific nutrients which enhance health*
2 *have been fortified with recognized nutrients such as vitamins*

3 *have been enriched with a nutrient or ingredient known to offer specific health benefits.*

For foods specifically marketed as a functional food, there should be scientific evidence of proven health benefits to support each product. Health claims should be based upon well-established evidence supported by scientific research literature, or recommendations from national or international public health bodies such as the Committee on Medical Aspects of Food and Nutrition Policy (COMA), the Food Standards Agency (FSA) or the US Food and Drug Administration (FDA).

PROBLEMS WITH FUNCTIONAL FOODS

There are a number of issues which make it difficult to know whether a functional food is really useful or not. For example:

▶ *Current legislation concentrates upon the safety of a product rather than the effectiveness of an added ingredient, so whilst an added ingredient may be safe to eat, it might not be adding any benefit.*
▶ *Health claims often relate to the active ingredient tested in isolation rather than in the product being bought.*
▶ *Some research stated on food packaging has been found to not actually relate to the added ingredient, but to a similar but different plant nutrient or strain of bacteria.*
▶ *Several foods in the UK and the USA have been withdrawn from the market for making unsubstantiated health claims on their food packaging.*

To help protect consumers from any misleading claims on foods, a new European Regulation came into force on 1 July 2007. Any claims made regarding the nutritional content or health benefits of a food will only be allowed if the claims are based on scientific evidence verified by the European Food Safety Authority (EFSA) and any claims made must be backed up by an explanation of how the active ingredient works. It will take time for all the health claims made to be reviewed, so it may be a while before you notice changes in the health claims made on food packaging.

Functional foods

Functional food	Added active ingredient and where it is naturally found	What the active ingredient does
Margarines or yoghurts	Phytosterols – plant sterols or plant stannols (*plant stannols are plant sterols that have been altered*) Found in vegetable oils, vegetables, fruits and grains	These compounds reduce cholesterol absorption in the digestive tract, hence reducing blood cholesterol levels.
Margarines, enriched eggs and juice	Omega 3 fatty acids Found in fish, linseeds, linseed oil, walnuts	Omega 3 fatty acids aid mental function, are an important structural component of cell membranes, reduce inflammation and help to counteract heart disease, strokes and cancer.
Yoghurts and yoghurt drinks	Probiotic bacteria and prebiotic plant fibres Probiotic bacteria are present in live yoghurt and prebiotic plant fibres are found in a range of fruit and vegetables	Lactic acid-forming bacteria create a healthy bowel environment, reducing the risk of yeast infections and bowel disease. Prebiotics are a type of indigestible fibre that provides food for healthy bowel flora.

Are functional foods useful?

Food manufacturers will always quote positive research about the active ingredient(s) in their product, but there are many elements that uphold or condemn research information. You probably won't be able to tell what type of research has been done by just reading a food label, but this may give you an idea as to how tenuous scientific evidence can be.

▶ *There should be a control group to compare results against in order to make sure the effects weren't due to a 'placebo effect'.*
▶ *Ideally, the product should have been tested on a significant number of people.*
▶ *The research should test the active ingredient once it has been added to the relevant functional food. Often, the research is based upon tests of the active ingredient itself, either in its natural format or in an isolated, concentrate form, not when it has been combined with its food 'host'.*

QUESTIONS TO ASK!

Q *Is there enough of the active ingredient present in the daily serving(s) to have an effect?*

Q *If you have to eat lots of the functional food to make its active ingredient effective, would this fit into a healthy diet?*

Q *Is the active ingredient still active?*

For example, the packaging on enriched margarines may promote the health benefits linked to the omega 3 fatty acids in their product, but there may be as little as 55 mg in two servings of margarine (enough for four slices of bread). A useful intake of omega 3 fatty acids is known to be approximately 1,000 mg (1 g) daily, which means you would have to eat enough margarine to spread on approximately 72 slices of bread every day... not a very healthy diet!

> **Insight: Try this instead**
> Instead of buying margarine enriched with small amounts of
> omega 3 fatty acids, just eat two portions of oily fish each week!

Laboratory studies have shown that probiotic drinks may improve
colon function and digestive health as long as the bacteria they
contain survive our stomach acid and digestion and reach the
colon, and if they can become established there. Many researchers
believe we would have to drink as much as 5 litres of probiotic
drinks daily to see any effect!

> **Insight: Try this instead**
> Instead of buying probiotic drinks, just choose live yoghurt,
> and ensure you eat five servings of fruit and vegetables a day
> for added prebiotics.

Benefits and drawbacks of functional foods

BENEFITS

Functional foods may be useful if a specific nutrient is low or
missing in your diet. For example, if you don't eat much fish or
linseeds/linseed oil in your diet, consuming foods with added
omega 3 fatty acids could be useful. This may be especially helpful
if these nutrients have been added to a food you normally eat,
increasing your intake of omega 3 fatty acids without having to
make lifestyle or dietary changes.

DRAWBACKS

However, although eating enriched foods seems an easy way to get
extra nutrients, consider these points before you fill up your trolley
with functional foods:

▶ *If the amount of the added nutrient is too low to be useful, you
may be better taking a probiotic or omega 3 supplement instead.*

- *The added nutrient may be denatured, unavailable or ineffective, as is often the case with added probiotics (live bacteria).*
- *Make sure that consuming functional foods isn't lulling you into a false sense of security, making you think you are consuming adequate and effective amounts of important nutrients when this may not be the case.*
- *If the functional food itself is not healthy, eating more of it to gain an added nutrient may be undermining the overall health of your diet.*

On that last point, eating large amounts of margarine, for example, is not necessarily the best way to consume phytosterols (plant sterols) to reduce cholesterol. Does it make sense to eat more margarine purely for the added plant compounds to help lower cholesterol? As elevated cholesterol levels often occur with increased body weight, this may not be the best way to lower cholesterol, as you would be simultaneously increasing your intake of fat and calories.

It has been suggested that health claims should be disallowed on foods that are...

- *high in fat (margarine, full fat yoghurts)*
- *high in salt (some breads and cereals)*
- *high in sugar (selected yoghurts, yoghurt drinks and some juices)*

... as these foods may have minimal nutritional value otherwise. It makes sense that a functional food should not be counterproductive to health despite its functional active ingredient.

So let's take a look at some of the specific active nutrients often added to our food, and consider whether you need more of this nutrient (there's little point buying a functional food otherwise!) and which functional or natural food source is the best option.

Omega 3 fatty acids

Over 200 new products enriched with omega 3 fatty acids were
added to the functional food market last year, with different
brands of juices, eggs, yoghurt and margarines strong favourites to
have this active ingredient added.

WHY ADD OMEGA 3 FATTY ACIDS TO FOOD?

As the only naturally rich sources of omega 3 fatty acids are fish,
algae and selected seeds (particularly linseeds), nuts and their
related oils, many people, especially non-fish eaters, struggle to
include enough of these essential fats in their diet. Whether we
need more omega 3 fats in our diet is not questionable: the vast
majority of people have eaten a diet rich in omega 6 fats (sunflower
oil, safflower oil and margarines) and low in omega 3 fats (fish and
linseeds) for a long period of time, creating a fatty acid imbalance.
Although a healthy diet should provide a ratio of approximately
3:1 (omega 6:omega 3), the average western diet has a fatty
acid ratio of approximately 16:1, so to correct a long-standing
imbalance, most of us need to consume more omega 3 fatty acids.

DO YOU NEED MORE OMEGA 3 FATTY ACIDS?

Although the vast majority of us would benefit from including
more omega 3 fats in our diet, our needs are all individual and

best assessed with the help of a registered nutritionist or dietician. However, there are some symptoms and health conditions that often respond well to an increased intake of polyunsaturated fats, particularly omega 3 fatty acids, indicating a potential deficiency. If you have any of the symptoms or conditions listed below, this may indicate a fatty acid deficiency or imbalance, particularly if your diet does not regularly include rich sources of omega 3 fatty acids.

Conditions that may indicate a fatty acid deficiency or imbalance:

- *eczema, asthma or hay fever*
- *skin conditions such as dermatitis or psoriasis*
- *inflammatory conditions such as colitis or arthritis*
- *poor concentration, poor memory function, learning difficulties*
- *anxiety or depression*
- *senile dementia and Alzheimer's Disease*
- *cardiovascular disease.*

If you suffer with one or more of these conditions, try to include more fish, linseeds, walnuts or enriched foods in your diet for a number of weeks and see if there are any improvements in your condition. Alternatively, consult your doctor or a qualified nutritionist for help, as many of these symptoms can also have other causes.

WHICH FOODS NATURALLY CONTAIN OMEGA 3 FATTY ACIDS?

- *Oily fish such as salmon, sardines, herring and pilchards.*
- *Linseeds (also known as flaxseed) and linseed oil.*
- *Some other oils and nuts such as rapeseed oil and walnuts.*
- *Green algae.*

WHAT DO OMEGA 3 FATTY ACIDS DO?

- *Omega 3 fatty acids have been linked with improved mental function.*
- *We need omega 3 fats to balance our inflammatory pathways.*

▶ *An adequate intake of omega 3 fats is linked with a reduced risk of stroke and heart disease.*
▶ *These fats maintain the flexibility and integrity of our cell membranes and artery walls.*

Insight: Note for non-fish eaters

Fish contain different fatty acids to the ones found in vegetable sources such linseeds, and although we can convert linolenic acid from these foods into the longer chain fats that have essential roles in mental and cardiovascular function, the conversion rate is very low. Conversion is impaired further with a high intake of omega 6 fatty acids from margarines and vegetable oils such as sunflower or safflower oil. Cut down on spreads, oils and saturated fats, and maybe try a fish oil supplement – check out Chapter 8 for more information on this subject.

So, although we only need the essential fatty acids in our diet (linolenic acid, an omega 3 fat, and linoleic acid, an omega 6 fat), if you are not adverse to fish oils, it's best to ensure a combination of fatty acids, including the longer chain fish oils, eicosapentanoic acid (EPA) and docosahexanoic acid (DHA), in your diet for full health benefits.

Although the simple answer is to eat more fish and linseeds rich in omega 3 fatty acids, functional foods enriched with omega 3 oils may give us the opportunity to continue with our normal diet and address this imbalance. Hence the appearance of enriched eggs, juices, margarines and yoghurts with added omega 3 fatty acids.

Insight: How to check what's been added to your food

If fish oils have been added to a food, the label should list eicosapentaenoic acid (EPA) and/or docosahexaenoic acid (DHA); if a vegetable source has been used the label will list linolenic acid or alpha-linolenic acid (LNA or ALA). This enables vegetarians and vegans to check which type of omega 3 fatty acid has been added to avoid inadvertently consuming fish oils.

Some food manufacturers struggle to hide the fishy smell or taste that comes from adding fish oils to their products so they use the vegetable source of linolenic acid instead. However, although this fat offers many known health benefits, much research linking reduced heart disease and improved mental function has been done specifically with the longer chain fish oils.

WHAT AMOUNT OF OMEGA 3 ACIDS DO I NEED?

It is worth ensuring that the amount of omega 3 fatty acids added to a food is likely to have a beneficial effect.

▶ *A recommended daily intake is 500 mg to 1 g, although some people with fatty acid deficiencies do benefit from more.*
▶ *One to two portions of fish a week would provide approximately 1–2 g of EPA and DHA.*
▶ *The UK Food Standards Agency (FSA) recommend that we eat two to four portions of fish a week, of which one to two portions should be oily fish.*

So if fish or other rich sources of omega 3 fatty acids are not present in your diet, you need at least 500 mg daily in your enriched diet. This table considers the omega 3 content of some enriched foods.

Omega 3 content of enriched foods

FOOD	How much do you need?	Is this healthy?
Enriched eggs	1 medium enriched egg provides approx. 600 mg EPA so you would need to eat 1–2 eggs daily.	Eggs are a healthy food, although they contain quite a lot of saturated fat and cholesterol. An egg a day could form part of a healthy diet.

(Contd)

FOOD	How much do you need?	Is this healthy?
Enriched juice	A 250 ml portion of juice may provide only 300 mg of ALA so you would have to drink 2–3 portions of juice daily. Some juices clearly market the health benefits of omega 3 fatty acids yet contain just a trace – not enough to be useful.	Avoid juices with added sugars and sweeteners. Don't forget that although ALA is an essential fatty acid the conversion rate into the longer chain fats linked with many additional health benefits may be less than 1%.
Enriched margarine	Some spreads provide only 55 mg of omega 3 fat in 20 g (enough for 3–4 slices of bread). You would need to eat almost ten times this amount to obtain the recommended omega 3 intake.	Increasing your intake of margarine spread would not be considered healthy.

If you rely on functional foods for your omega 3 fatty acids, a healthier option is to eat a number of enriched foods rather than eating too much of any one food. Here's an example of an omega 3 enriched day:

Breakfast	Enriched eggs on wholemeal toast with enriched spread
Snack	Omega 3 enriched yoghurt
Lunch	Salad sandwich with omega 3 enriched juice
Snack	Linseed and walnut bar and glass of enriched juice
Dinner	Follow meat/fish or nut roast with an enriched yoghurt

CONSIDERING THE BEST OPTION FOR OMEGA 3 FATTY ACIDS – ENRICHED EGGS

Hens fed a diet that is fortified with omega 3 fatty acids sourced from algae, fish or linseeds will produce eggs that contain higher levels of omega 3 fats, as shown in this table. These values are based upon hens fed ten per cent flaxseed in the diet and values are for one egg.

Omega 3 enriched eggs

	Omega 3 enriched egg	Normal egg
Total fats	4.9 g	5 g
Omega 6 fats	0.7 g	0.7 g
Omega 3 fats	0.4 g	0.04 g
Monounsaturated fats	1.6 g	2 g
Saturated fats	1.2 g	1.5 g
Cholesterol	185 mg	190 mg

Information from the Canadian Egg Marketing Agency, 2007.

This illustrates the differences between a standard and an enriched egg, although other brands of eggs will have a different fatty acid profile. Columbus enriched eggs contain twice as many omega 3 fats at 0.85 g (850 mg) per egg, helping you to achieve the intake recommended in the Scientific Advisory Committee on Nutrition Report (2006) of 0.45 g (450 mg) of omega 3 fatty acids every day. The actual levels of omega 3 and omega 6 fats should be shown on egg boxes.

Will eating enriched eggs have the desired effect?
An extra millimole per litre (mmol/L) in blood triglyceride levels can increase the risk of heart disease by 76 per cent in women and 32 per cent in men; including enriched eggs in the diet has been shown to decrease blood triglyceride levels. However, some studies show slightly elevated cholesterol levels from consuming extra eggs

(normal and enriched), and elevated cholesterol is a risk factor for coronary heart disease. Further studies have shown elevated levels of 'good' HDL cholesterol after eating omega 3 enriched eggs, which helps to reduce 'bad' and overall cholesterol levels. Although the cholesterol in eggs seems to have little effect upon our cholesterol levels, consuming saturated fat (also present in eggs) does have a detrimental effect upon cholesterol levels.

Benefits and drawbacks of consuming enriched eggs

▶ *As part of a healthy diet, enriched eggs can increase your intake of omega 3 fats.*
▶ *Enriched eggs may also have a healthier fatty acid profile, containing less saturated fat and cholesterol than a normal egg.*

However ...

▶ *Eggs are still a source of cholesterol and saturated fat and consumption should be limited because of this, particularly if the diet contains full-fat dairy products and meat, which also contain saturated fats.*

The final verdict on enriched eggs:

▶ *Swap to enriched eggs for a better fatty acid profile.*
▶ *Choose organic and free range whenever possible.*
▶ *Don't eat more eggs, just enjoy the benefits of the enriched version.*
▶ *Obtain omega 3 fatty acids from other foods such as fish and seeds.*

Back to nature

Although eggs are much more nutritious than many functional foods and provide a healthy way to obtain extra omega 3 fatty acids, fish consumption has been linked with several health benefits, including lower cholesterol levels, suggesting that eating foods naturally rich in omega 3 fatty acids is the best way to obtain this nutrient.

Insight: The best source of EPA and DHA...

For the highest levels of EPA and DHA in fish, eat wild or organically farmed fish. Fatty acids are in the algae which wild fish eat, whilst farmed fish are often fed synthetic food with a lower concentration of omega 3 fatty acids. Organically farmed fish are fed recycled fish and shellfish already caught for human consumption rather than synthetic food, so are likely to consume more omega 3 fatty acids than other farmed fish.

Plant sterols

One of the most well known functional foods is the plant sterol- or phytosterol-enriched margarine spread. Tests have shown that plant sterols can reduce LDL or 'bad' cholesterol; however, we need to consume 2–3 g of plant sterols daily to achieve this. If your intake of plant sterols is coming from functional foods, you'll have to consume a specific amount of these enriched products daily. Let's consider the fortified spreads...

DO YOU NEED MORE PLANT STEROLS IN YOUR DIET?

Studies have shown that plant sterols added to foods are most helpful in reducing existing high cholesterol levels in contrast to preventing elevated cholesterol.

Insight

You may benefit from more phytosterols in your diet if your total cholesterol is over 5 mmol/l, or you have LDL ('bad' cholesterol) of over 2.6 mmol/l.

Eating more phytosterol-enriched foods will be even more effective if you make the following changes to your diet.

WAYS TO HELP REDUCE CHOLESTEROL WITH A NORMAL HEALTHY DIET

1 *Decrease your intake of saturated fat by reducing your intake of full-fat dairy foods, eggs, meats and bakery products such as biscuits and cakes.*
2 *Swap butter for a spread enriched with plant sterols.*
3 *Swap full-fat yoghurts for lower fat, phytosterol-enriched yoghurts.*
4 *Choose low-fat milk also enriched with plant sterols.*
5 *Eat plenty of fibrous fruit, vegetables, oats and beans which also help to reduce the amount of circulating cholesterol in the body.*

We would all benefit from eating more vegetables rich in soluble fibre, because this type of fibre promotes good health in many ways. In addition to reducing cholesterol levels, plant fibres have been proven to:

▶ *improve food peristalsis along the gut and reduce constipation*
▶ *help regulate glucose absorption and blood sugar control*
▶ *improve bowel flora and function*
▶ *increase satiety and help weight control.*

> **Insight: Other tips to lower cholesterol levels**
> ✓ *Eat more fish.*
> ✓ *Include soya products in your diet.*
> ✓ *Include nuts in your diet.*

ARE ENRICHED SPREADS HEALTHY?

You may be able to reduce your cholesterol levels by regularly consuming a spread enriched with plant sterols, but it's worth checking whether your chosen spread also contains trans or hydrogenated fatty acids, which are two types of fat to avoid as they are detrimental to health. You could be reducing your risk of heart disease by lowering cholesterol on one hand, but simultaneously increasing your risk by consuming trans or hydrogenated fats!

The amount of enriched margarine spread that one leading manufacturer suggests is needed daily to provide cholesterol lowering effects is 25 g. This would provide over 100 calories daily. If you are concerned about your weight, can you afford to consume the additional fat and calories every day, especially when the food only conveys a benefit that could equally be gained through eating low-calorie, high-fibre fruit and vegetables? You weigh it up! Even the product manufacturers state that to add this amount of fat to your diet and still achieve weight loss, the extra calories in the margarine spread must be offset with a calorie reduction elsewhere.

HOW EFFECTIVE ARE PLANT STEROLS AT REDUCING CHOLESTEROL?

Plant sterols have been repeatedly proven to lower overall and low density lipoprotein (LDL or 'bad') cholesterol; however, better results have been obtained by combining sterol-enriched foods with a healthier diet as follows:

Cholesterol reduction

Reduction in cholesterol from using margarines with plant sterols added	Reduction in cholesterol from using enriched margarines PLUS eating more vegetables, fruit, soya and nuts
TOTAL CHOLESTEROL ↓ 10%	TOTAL CHOLESTEROL ↓ 22.34%
LDL CHOLESTEROL ↓ 14%	LDL CHOLESTEROL ↓ 29.71%

(Buckley et al., 2007. The Journal of Family Practice, Vol. 56 (1).)

When you consider that these reductions in cholesterol remain only as long as the dietary adjustment continues, how you choose to reduce your cholesterol has to be sustainable – and good for overall health in the long run. In short, you could get the same results from following a healthy Mediterranean-style diet, whilst simultaneously enjoying several additional health benefits that this type of diet provides.

Gemma swapped a diet of pastries, burgers, crisps and sweets for a healthy diet rich in fruit, vegetables, fish and whole grains to lose weight. Not only did she lose a stone over six weeks, but her cholesterol reduced from 7.4 mmol/L to 5.1 mmol/L.

A DOWNSIDE TO PLANT STEROLS

Although plant sterols have been proven to lower cholesterol, they can also reduce carotenoid levels by seven per cent or more. Carotenoids are anti-oxidants that fight cell damage, support immune function and reduce the effects of ageing (See Chapter 3 and Chapter 6 for more information about these natural phytonutrients). In trying to reduce cholesterol levels by consuming extra plant sterols in enriched foods, we may inadvertently create another problem.

Insight
The National Heart Foundation in Australia has recommended a limited consumption of added plant sterols or stanols and advised eating at least one serving of carotenoid-rich foods daily to maintain carotene levels for those consuming plant sterol enriched foods.

Carotenoid-rich foods
- *Carrots*
- *Sweet potato*
- *Squash and pumpkin*
- *Peaches and apricots*

This problem doesn't happen to the same extent when we consume a natural, healthy diet, which questions whether it is wiser to simply consume more fruit and vegetables naturally containing plant fibre and sterols (and carotenoids!) in order to reduce cholesterol. In fact, a healthy consumption of plant foods is likely to have prevented an increase in cholesterol levels in the first place.

Do functional foods cost more?

A margarine spread with added plant sterols may cost over £2 more for a 500 g tub, so the simple answer is 'yes'! You aren't exactly getting something for nothing! A suggested intake of functional foods to consume the required amount of sterols every week is shown opposite.

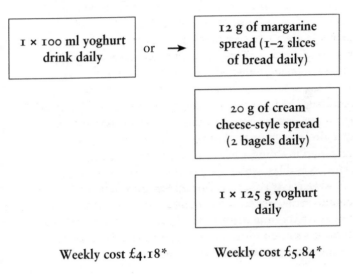

| 1 × 100 ml yoghurt drink daily | or → | 12 g of margarine spread (1–2 slices of bread daily) |

20 g of cream cheese-style spread (2 bagels daily)

1 × 125 g yoghurt daily

Weekly cost £4.18*   Weekly cost £5.84*

*prices correct at time of publication

A direct comparison with the cost of getting your plant sterols and cholesterol-lowering fibre from vegetables looks reasonable, as five servings of vegetables a day could cost £9.24 over a week. However, we still need to eat vegetables for vitamins, minerals, energy, fibre and fluid as well as the rich variety of phytonutrients (see Chapter 3), so although having an enriched yoghurt drink daily may seem less expensive unless you plan to forego fruit and vegetables altogether, this doesn't represent a saving at all.

In fact, relying on functional foods to provide one specific nutrient (in this case plant sterols) could turn out to be an expensive mistake for your health. Fruits and vegetables have been proven to have the following beneficial effects upon health:

1 *lowering cholesterol*
2 *decreasing constipation, haemorrhoids and diverticulosis*
3 *providing indigestible prebiotic plant fibres for enhanced gut flora*
4 *decreasing blood pressure and the risk of heart disease*
5 *decreasing the risk of cancer*
6 *supporting immune function with anti-oxidant nutrients*
7 *support of detoxification processes*
8 *anti-bacterial, anti-viral activity*
9 *improved control of hormones and hormone metabolism*
10 *enhanced weight management.*

The sterol-enriched functional food can be a useful, if expensive, adjunct to any diet, as it adds an additional amount of plant sterols to your daily consumption, but you will never gain all of the benefits found in eating a selection (five servings or more a day) of fruits and vegetables, which would simultaneously help to lower cholesterol levels. If you are choosing functional foods for health purposes, the comparison between an enriched product containing plant sterols and eating plant foods illustrates the obvious choice. See Chapter 3 to see how a diet rich in natural phytosterols and inulin plant fibre can lower your cholesterol.

The probiotic and prebiotic revolution

Although 'live' yoghurts have been around for a while, one of our most popular functional foods are those with added pre- and probiotics. Probiotic means 'for life', and relates to the healthy bacteria that can exert a beneficial effect in our gut. These bacteria are those that, in health, normally inhabit our bowel and have several roles in maintaining health:

▶ *They affect the pH (acidity or alkalinity) to create an optimum environment.*

- *They help to prevent strains of unhealthy bacteria and fungi from growing (such as Clostridium and Candida).*
- *Healthy bowel florae promote the synthesis and absorption of vitamins such as vitamin K and several B vitamins.*
- *A healthy gut promotes the absorption of minerals like iron and calcium.*
- *With good colonic health we naturally produce antibiotic-like substances to inhibit the overgrowth and colonization of fungal, bacterial and viral organisms, including 'travel bugs'.*

Previously unknown strains of 'friendly bacteria' are constantly being discovered and it's true that we all have our own unique 'flora footprint' with differing concentrations of microbes in each individual, but the two most well-known strains of healthy gut bacteria are:

- *Lactobacillus species (for example, Lactobacillus acidophilus)*
- *Bifidobacterium species (for example, Bifidobacterium bifidum).*

DO YOU NEED PROBIOTICS?

Owing to our typical westernized diet, rich in meats, dairy produce, sugars and refined carbohydrates and generally deficient in fruit and vegetables, most of us would benefit from a good probiotic. If this describes your usual diet, the chances are that your bowel flora is not ideal and a probiotic food or supplement may help re-create a better environment in your gut. However, this will be of little use if you continue to consume a diet that is high in protein, sugar and refined carbohydrates and low in fruit and vegetables.

If you regularly suffer with the following symptoms, which are indications of putrefactive (bad) bowel bacteria and dysbiosis (disturbed/unhealthy bowel flora), a probiotic may help – as long as it is an effective product.

Symptoms of dysbiosis:

- *flatulence*
- *diarrhoea*

- *constipation*
- *foul-smelling stools*
- *bowel cramps*
- *irregular bowel movements*
- *thrush*
- *yeast infections such as athlete's foot or yeast in the mouth*
- *severe fatigue*
- *food allergies*
- *headaches.*

In a healthy gut, the 'good' bacteria normally keep unhealthy organisms in check; this helps to avoid bowel conditions which can ultimately lead to irritable bowel syndrome, yeast infections such as candidiasis, ulcerative colitis, haemorroids, diverticular disease and colon cancer.

Several lifestyle and dietary habits can reduce the levels of healthy bacteria in our bowel, affecting the delicate balance of flora. The most common culprits are listed below.

- *antibiotics*
- *long-term use of the contraceptive pill*
- *steroids (for example, cortisone, HRT)*
- *smoking*
- *stress*
- *eating large amounts of meat and dairy produce, or consuming a diet high in protein*
- *eating large amounts of sugars and refined carbohydrates such as bread, biscuits, cakes, etc.*
- *regular alcohol consumption*
- *lack of dietary fibre found in fruits and vegetables.*

If you can hold your hands up to more than one of these, the chances are that your bowel flora – the type of bacteria in your bowel – is not as healthy as it could be!

Bad bacteria thrive in the type of colonic environment created by high intakes of sugars, processed carbohydrates and eating too much protein food. Considering our typical diet, you can see how the environment in our bowels can easily become hostile to friendly bacteria and can encourage the growth of unhealthy bacteria! Once the unhealthy bacteria have grown in numbers, a battle between the 'good' and 'bad' bacteria determines which strains of flora inhabit the gut. Furthermore, the bacterial strains in the highest numbers create the colonic environment to suit their own growth and counteract further growth of the competing bacteria.

DO PROBIOTIC FUNCTIONAL FOODS WORK?

There have been several criticisms of probiotics:

1 *The number of bacteria in the product may be too low to have any significant effect. This may be due to the number of flora in the product to begin with or too many bacteria not surviving production and storage methods, so by the time you consume the probiotic there may be very few viable organisms present.*
2 *The bacteria have to be able to withstand the stomach and bile acids in the digestive tract to reach the target destination of the colon and many strains included in probiotic foods do not survive digestion.*
3 *Strains of bacteria should always be those found in the large intestine in health, for example, Lactobacillus acidophilus or Bifidobacterium bifidum.*

How many bacteria are needed to be effective?
To ensure that a viable number of organisms are still available when a product is consumed, several billion organisms need to be added. For example, a typical bowel flora supplement might contain up to 24 billion active bacteria in one dose and probiotic drinks may state that 6.5–10 billion bacteria have been added to each drink. However, studies have repeatedly shown that the numbers of bacteria in many commercial probiotic products is significantly lower than that stated.

Will the bacteria survive digestion?

The bacteria must either be a resistant strain, be in a milk product
or in a coated capsule that provides protection against the digestive
processes in the gut. Again, in independent research, most bacterial
strains present in probiotic products failed to withstand the
digestive processes, although certain Lactobacillus strains were
most successful in surviving. However, those that did survive the
digestive process seemed to have little effect upon the colonic
microflora of the large intestine.

What should I look for in a probiotic?

▶ *Look for the Lactobacillus and Bifidobacterium species in
  significant numbers.*
▶ *Choose dairy products, particularly fermented milk products –
  these increase the effectiveness of probiotics as they offer some
  protection against the digestive processes.*
▶ *Fermented milk products also provide food for the bacteria to
  grow and feed upon during storage and digestion.*
▶ *Lactic acid bacteria thrive when indigestible plant fibre is
  present, so a product with added prebiotics is a bonus. These
  products are also known as synbiotics, due to the synergistic
  relationship between the bacteria (probiotics) and the
  indigestible plant fibre (prebiotics).*
▶ *The prebiotics also enhance the colonic environment, helping
  the healthy bacteria to grow in the gut and continue to inhabit
  it for a longer period.*
▶ *Avoid using probiotic products with added sugar as this will
  largely reverse any health benefits gained from increasing
  the number of probiotic bacteria in your bowel, as it creates
  adverse conditions for the 'good' bacteria to survive in.*

There is little point in consuming probiotics to improve bowel health whilst continuing to create unhealthy bowel conditions – any bacteria which manage to inhabit the bowel will have a very short stay if conditions are unfavourable – try following Level 2 of the detox diet in Chapter 4 for a bowel-healthy diet!

PREBIOTICS

A prebiotic is a name for the food or substrate that the healthy bacteria live off in the bowel. Prebiotics are generally different types of fibre found in fruits and vegetables, and a fibre called inulin is one of the most effective prebiotics. As most fibre isn't digested, it continues through the digestive tract to the large intestine and colon, where it provides food for the bacteria and creates the right environment in the bowel for healthy bacteria to live in.

Foods rich in inulin
▶ *Chicory (a salad leaf)*
▶ *Jerusalem artichokes*
▶ *Asparagus*
▶ *Onions*
▶ *Garlic.*

Insight: A good idea

A good probiotic supplement from a reputable company rather than a functional food is more likely to deliver the right strain and required number of bacteria to the gut. Contained within coated capsules to ensure resistance to stomach and bile acid digestion, some supplements release each bacterial strain in the part of the gut that it normally inhabits, with none of the added sugar found in probiotic functional foods. Many supplements also contain prebiotics.

Will functional foods work for you?

In short, functional foods do sometimes provide us with that little bit extra, but often at our expense. If you are buying the food anyway, enjoy the added benefits, but don't be mislead into thinking you are following a healthy diet if you haven't got the basics covered.

Remember, the basics are:

- *five servings of fruit and vegetables daily*
- *at least eight large glasses of water*
- *wholegrain, starchy carbohydrates and protein foods in each meal*
- *a good intake of essential fatty acids from fish, seeds, nuts and oils.*

All functional foods should be healthy foods in their own right in order to really contribute to a healthy diet.

There are several considerations to be made in order to decide whether the functional food is right for you:

- *Time*
- *Budget*
- *Lifestyle.*

The ideal scenario will always be to consume a healthy balanced diet full of fresh foods, which will automatically help to create a healthy environment in the gut, keep cholesterol levels in check, and provide the essential fatty acids needed for health.

However, if you dislike fish and seeds, eat few vegetables and follow a lifestyle that leaves little option to choose low-sugar, high-fibre foods on a daily basis, then some functional foods may help. But consider these points before you fill up your supermarket trolley:

- *Would it really take so long to open a bag of prepared salad?*
- *Is it so difficult to grab a piece of fruit?*
- *Why can't you choose a salmon or mackerel salad sandwich rather than meat or cheese?*
- *Why not try adding seeds to yoghurts, stir fries and cereals?*

It's essential not to rely on functional foods alone for health, when the wealth of benefits from including more fruit, vegetables, fish and seeds in your diet is fairly impressive:

▶ *Improved bowel function*
▶ *Reduced risk of diverticulosis*
▶ *Reduced risk of haemorrhoids*
▶ *Reduced risk of colorectal cancer and some other cancers*
▶ *Reduced risk of stroke and heart disease*
▶ *Lower blood pressure*
▶ *Reduced cholesterol levels*
▶ *Enhanced immune function*
▶ *Improved eye health*
▶ *Lower body weight*
▶ *Fewer inflammatory reactions*
▶ *Enhanced mental function*
▶ *Reduced cellular damage resulting in less ageing.*

You don't see a list of benefits like that on a so-called functional food! The choice is yours!

THINGS TO REMEMBER

If you do like the idea of functional foods, remember to choose wisely...

- *What does the food contain that provides a health benefit – and do you need it? If you already eat fish three or four times weekly, you may not need omega-3 fortified foods.*

- *Make sure you're happy to consume the added nutrient – vegetarians and vegans will not want to consume vegetable-based foods with added fish oils to boost their omega-3 intake. Non-fish eaters should look for ALA or LNA rather than EPA and DHA on the added ingredients list.*

- *Does it contain the active nutrient in high enough levels to be effective? This is particularly important for probiotics.*

- *Are you happy to continue including the functional food in your diet? Checking information such as calorie and fat content may be worthwhile if you are watching your weight.*

... and above all else, don't rely on functional foods in place of a nutritious diet for good health.

6

How to look (and be!) younger

In this chapter you will learn:
- *what causes ageing*
- *how you can reduce ageing*
- *what an anti-ageing diet consists of.*

We all want to look and feel our best and the saying 'you are what you eat' is no truer than in this context. Our body is made up of the very foods we consume and the way that we look and feel is a direct result of our diet. In our increasingly developed society it has become more difficult to maintain a healthy diet rich in the nutrients we require for health and longevity. With increased pollution, over-farmed nutrient-poor soils, higher levels of stress and increased exposure to solar radiation, our requirement for nutrients has increased as our intake has decreased owing to a largely processed diet. However, there are many simple ways to increase our nutrient intake and get older without 'ageing'!

Anti-ageing smoothie!

Get started on your anti-ageing regime straight away with this smoothie packed with anti-oxidants. Blend a cup of blueberries, a cup of strawberries and a cup of raspberries with a cup of soya milk. For a thicker consistency add a spoonful of live yoghurt or a ripe banana.
DONE!

What is ageing?

There are several theories as to how and why we age – here are the most common:

- ▶ *pre-programmed biological timetables*
- ▶ *as a result of environmental assault*
- ▶ *a timed switching on and off certain genes which regulate cell renewal.*

What seems to be generally agreed is that our lifespan is determined by our genetics in conjunction with our lifestyle, the latter causing wear and tear, protein alterations and free radical damage.

:..:
: GENETICS + LIFESTYLE = RATE OF AGEING   :
:..:

Although there seem to be many different ways in which we age, there is a common denominator that causes these changes as we become older. This common cause is cellular damage. Whether the damage is done to our skin, giving us wrinkles, to our arteries, causing atherosclerosis, or to our pancreas, causing diabetes, if we can reduce the cellular damage, we can reduce, prevent or even partially reverse some of the ageing process.

There are many symptoms of ageing, but here are some of the more well-known conditions we associate with getting older:

- ▶ *skin damage – wrinkles, thinner skin, liver spots, loss of elasticity*
- ▶ *obesity and loss of body shape, less lean tissue*
- ▶ *heart disease – elevated blood pressure and cholesterol levels, atherosclerosis (fatty deposits in the arteries), arteriosclerosis (hardening of the arteries), thrombosis, stroke and heart attack*
- ▶ *diabetes*
- ▶ *arthritis, osteoporosis and joint problems*
- ▶ *immune decline leading to lower resistance to infection*
- ▶ *poor digestion, diverticulitis, bowel disease and cancer*

- *impaired mental function – loss of memory, reduced cognitive function*
- *nerve damage leading to Parkinson's disease and other disorders*
- *eye problems – macular degeneration, cataracts and glaucoma.*

Although all of these conditions affect different organs and systems, apart from disease that may have targeted a particular organ, much of the damage that causes these conditions is a build up of cellular damage, commonly known as 'wear and tear'. One of the most common causes of cellular damage is oxidative free radicals.

Free radicals (unstable molecules or atoms) are a natural occurrence. They are produced by every cell in the body, our immune system uses them to kill bacteria and they are also used in nerve cells. However, constant bombardment from free radicals eventually destroys cells unless the damage is repaired, causing common signs of wear and tear, or ageing.

EXAMPLES OF CELLULAR FREE RADICAL DAMAGE

- *Cells may not be able to produce enough cartilage to protect our joints, which would lead to osteoarthritis.*
- *We may no longer produce enough collagen to keep our skin soft and supple, resulting in sagging skin and wrinkles.*
- *Our arteries may become less flexible, creating higher blood pressure and increasing the risk of atherosclerosis.*

Hence, symptoms of 'ageing' appear as oxidative damage accumulates. In fact, some experts state that up to 80–90 per cent of disease is due to free radical damage!

Anti-oxidants are our main source of protection against free radical damage. There are several variables which affect the rate at which we age and the amount of anti-oxidants in our diet is just one of these variables, but it is one element that we have some control over! Although research into how much effect an anti-oxidant rich diet or supplementing with anti-oxidants can have upon the ageing process is lacking, it is known that certain anti-oxidants can reduce the risk of cataracts, cancer, heart disease and diabetes, so a healthy, anti-oxidant rich diet will definitely affect at least some of the symptoms of old age, even if it doesn't actually stop our biological clock!

What determines how much free radical damage you have?
Free radicals are present everywhere – in our bodies, in the environment and in some of the foods we eat. The trick is to minimize free radical damage by firstly reducing our exposure to it and also boosting our intake of protective anti-oxidants.

Free radicals may come from…
- *Exposure to sunlight or UV light (for example, sun beds)*
- *Pollution*
- *Smoking*
- *Radiation*
- *Carcinogens (substances which alter cellular DNA and cause cancer)*
- *Heated oils which have become unstable*
- *Polyunsaturated oils exposed to light/sunlight.*

These can be 'quenched' or neutralized by anti-oxidants such as these…
- ✓ *Vitamin C*
- ✓ *Vitamin E*
- ✓ *Beta carotene*
- ✓ *Zinc (an anti-oxidant mineral)*
- ✓ *Selenium (another anti-oxidant mineral).*

The rate at which we age is affected by our genetics and our lifestyle. If you live in a city where air pollution is higher, you have smoked for a number of years and enjoy sunbathing, you are exposing yourself to more free radicals than a non-smoker who lives in the countryside and avoids sunbathing! However, we also have individual requirements for nutrients; some of us can absorb anti-oxidant nutrients easily, and may need less in the diet to counteract the free radical damage which causes us to age.

Another way in which we neutralize free radicals and potential carcinogens is through our detoxification system which is primarily in our liver (see Chapter 4 for more information on detoxification). Ensuring that we have sufficient nutrients for effective detoxification will also help us to avoid unnecessary cellular damage. Again, the anti-oxidants are required for this process, but vegetables such as onions, garlic, broccoli, cauliflower and cabbage also provide essential nutrients needed for detoxification.

Top ten anti-ageing diet tips

Stopping smoking, limiting exposure to pollution and using sunscreen will all help to limit free radical damage. But in order to reduce, prevent, and maybe even reverse (as our cells are being renewed continuously) the cellular damage that causes ageing, here's how you should adjust your diet:

1 *Limit your calorie intake!*
2 *Eat an anti-oxidant rich diet (this means eating 'five a day').*
3 *Include foods that will limit free radical damage.*
4 *Avoid the 'bad' fats (saturated fat, hydrogenated and trans fatty acids and cholesterol).*
5 *Cook with olive oil.*
6 *Fill up on the good fats.*
7 *Limit oxidative damage to fats.*
8 *Limit your intake of substances that can cause free radical damage.*
9 *Reduce your intake of sugar and refined carbohydrates.*
10 *Limit your alcohol intake and choose heart-healthy red wine.*

Let's take a look at each of these anti-ageing tips in more detail.

1 CALORIE RESTRICTION TO STAY YOUNG?

Animal research has shown that calorie restriction reduces or slows the ageing process, prolonging life expectancy by one third to twice as long as expected.

How does it work?

Excess weight contributes to diabetes, heart disease and some cancers, puts additional pressure on our joints, and increases inflammation and cell damage, contributing to ageing in many different ways. Metabolizing food energy creates free radicals, so lowering food intake reduces free radical formation.

2 EAT AN ANTI-OXIDANT RICH DIET

This is one of the most important things you can do to limit ageing and prevent disease. Fruit and vegetables are naturally rich in anti-oxidants; they will not contain trans and hydrogenated fats; and they are low-calorie foods, so including these in your diet has several anti-ageing benefits.

For an anti-oxidant fix eat this every day

Bionic salad!

Mix these ingredients together for an anti-oxidant fix: avocado, a selection of watercress, rocket, and spinach leaves, vine tomatoes, grated carrot, diced beetroot, sliced peppers, sweetcorn and red onion. Drizzle with salad dressing – olive oil or linseed oil with chopped chillies, grated garlic and a squeeze of lemon juice.

Which foods have the highest anti-oxidant content?
A 'score' for anti-oxidant power has been formulated in the USA. It is called ORAC (Oxygen Radical Absorbance Capacity). It measures the anti-oxidant power of foods and herbs, which indicates the amount of free radicals that an anti-oxidant can neutralize. Findings from the USDA (United States Department of Agriculture) suggest that we can help to slow down the ageing process by eating a diet rich in foods that have a high ORAC score.

Foods with the highest ORAC anti-oxidant power

Food	ORAC units per 100 g
Prunes	5,770
Raisins	2,830
Blueberries	2,400
Blackberries	2,036
Kale	1,770
Strawberries	1,540
Spinach	1,260
Raspberries	1,220
Brussels sprouts	980
Alfalfa sprouts	930
Broccoli	890

The foods that have the highest anti-oxidant score are the fruits and vegetables, particularly berries, green vegetables and orange-coloured fruit and vegetables rich in beta carotene. You can find other anti-oxidants such as zinc and selenium in whole grains, nuts, seeds, meat and seafood (especially oysters).

3 LIMIT FREE RADICAL DAMAGE

Our detoxification system requires several nutrients found in garlic, onions, green leafy vegetables and protein foods, as well as the anti-oxidants already discussed. These foods should be included in your diet every day.

- ✓ *Garlic – eat two cloves every day.*
- ✓ *Onions – eat one medium-sized onion daily.*
- ✓ *Broccoli, sprouts, cauliflower or cabbage – eat at least one serving daily.*
- ✓ *Beta carotene-rich foods – eat at least one serving daily.*
- ✓ *Protein foods – eating fish, soya and eggs will provide the final ingredients that enable your liver to detoxify and limit free radical damage.*

Cruciferous vegetables such as broccoli contain iron and manganese as well as compounds known as thiols which are all essential to the detoxification process. Dark green vegetables are also rich in anti-oxidants beta carotene and vitamin C, making this group of foods a must-have in your detoxification, anti-ageing menu!

4 AVOID THE 'BAD' FATS

A high intake of saturated fat is connected with many diseases that occur more frequently as we age:

▶ *heart disease*
▶ *elevated cholesterol*
▶ *elevated blood pressure*
▶ *fatty liver*
▶ *obesity*
▶ *some cancers.*

These types of fats are found predominantly in animal meats, eggs and full-fat dairy products, as well as cakes and pastries. However, organically reared poultry and animals provide a better quality of meat, eggs and milk with a healthier ratio of fatty acids; together with the many minerals and vitamins these foods provide, they can contribute to a healthy diet if not eaten in excess. The refined and saturated fats found in foods such as pastry, cakes and biscuits, however, do not convey any health benefits, so this is a good place to start if you need to reduce your fat intake.

Do you need to limit cholesterol intake?

Dietary cholesterol does not significantly affect cholesterol levels: in health, the more cholesterol we consume, the less our liver produces, so the amount of cholesterol circulating in our body is maintained within normal limits. Hypercholesterolaemia is often due to genetically elevated cholesterol levels, or liver dysfunction, as the liver continues to produce cholesterol despite elevated blood cholesterol levels.

However, it makes sense to limit high-cholesterol foods such as eggs, some shellfish and full-fat dairy foods, as the additional cholesterol is not required, and these foods are also high in saturated fat which can elevate cholesterol levels.

Insight: Did you know?

Hydrogenated fats are polyunsaturated fats that have been turned into manufactured saturated fats, with all the negative health implications saturated fats are associated with.

This is how margarines made with vegetable oils, which should be liquid at room temperature, are actually solid and spreadable – they've been turned into saturated fats, which are solid at room temperature!

Many similar products also contain partially hydrogenated vegetable oils, where the fatty acids have not been completely hydrogenated (saturated) but trans fats may have been formed during the process. Partially hydrogenated fats are often used in processed foods to:

▶ *create certain food textures*
▶ *improve food palatability*
▶ *form spreadable products*
▶ *increase shelf life.*

Hydrogenated and partially hydrogenated fats are found in margarines, sauces, gravy mixes, salad dressings and refined bakery goods, and also in sweets, chocolate and French fries.

Why avoid them?

▶ *Hydrogenation destroys the beneficial essential fatty acids, replacing them with toxic fatty substances.*
▶ *Trans fats that are taken up into the tissues contribute to elevated cholesterol levels, atherosclerosis and heart disease.*
▶ *They also interfere with the essential roles of healthy fatty acids and can affect immune function, insulin control and reduce the effectiveness of liver enzymes responsible for detoxification.*
▶ *There is also a close correlation between the amount of trans fat consumed and cancer occurrence.*

In contrast to the damage that these processed fats cause, the essential fatty acids have been shown to reverse the effects of hydrogenated and trans fatty acids.

5 COOK WITH OLIVE OIL

Olive oil is well known as being one of the foods in the healthy Mediterranean-style diet. It is one of the healthiest oils to cook with, as it is neither saturated nor polyunsaturated. Saturated fats such as lard or butter will not become oxidized during cooking but may contribute to atherosclerosis (fatty deposits in the arteries). In contrast, the molecular structure of polyunsaturated oils such as safflower and sunflower increases the risk of oxidization during heating. Oxidization is when oxygen atoms attach to the oil, but become loose after consumption, turning into free radicals and causing cellular damage.

Insight: Olive oil benefits

Olive oil is made up of mostly mono-unsaturated fatty acids, so less oxidative damage can occur during heating. Swap your polyunsaturated sunflower or safflower oils to olive oil to reduce free radical damage from oxidized fats. It is this quality that is thought to contribute to the cardio-protective benefits of the Mediterranean diet.

6 FILL UP ON THE GOOD FATS!

Not all fats are bad; in fact, some are a necessity for good health. Fats should provide between 15–30 per cent of our daily caloric intake and this should come from fish, nuts, seeds and natural oils, with a limited amount of fat from lean meats, eggs, shellfish and dairy produce. Increased consumption of fish, nuts, seeds and vegetable oils has been connected with the following health benefits:

✓ *Reduced risk of heart disease.*
✓ *Improved mood and behaviour.*
✓ *Reduced cholesterol levels.*

✓ *Lower blood pressure.*
✓ *Improved blood glucose control.*
✓ *Fewer inflammatory diseases.*
✓ *Reduced incidence of allergies.*
✓ *Better gastrointestinal health and bowel motility.*
✓ *Improved immune function.*
✓ *Reduced incidence of cancer.*
✓ *Improved mental function.*

Considering that several diseases commonly associated with ageing can be improved with a balanced intake of omega 3 fatty acids, this is an essential part of an 'anti-ageing' diet.

Foods rich in the good fats
✓ *Fish*
✓ *Nuts*
✓ *Seeds*
✓ *Avocados.*

Fill up on fish with these ideas!

Breakfast	Kippers or kedgeree (see recipe in Chapter 3, page 85)
Lunch	Sardines on toast
Dinner	Baked salmon steak with vegetables
Snacks	Peppered mackerel on crisp breads or Ryvita

Veggie menu!

Breakfast	An omega 3 enriched egg or fruit smoothie with linseeds
Lunch	Avocado on seeded bread toasted with a mixed green leaf and walnut salad with linseed oil dressing
Dinner	Vegetable stir fry with added seeds, drizzled with linseed oil
Snacks	Seed/nut bar

Essential fatty acids regulate inflammation, cell membrane flexibility, movement of cellular substances and nerve transmission to name just a few functions, so it's easy to see how a deficiency or imbalance causes symptoms of ill health or disease. Lack of the 'good' fats in the diet can cause the following problems – tick any that apply to you, and if you have just one or two ticks, increase your intake of fish or seeds!

Dry skin	☐
Eczema	☐
Asthma	☐
Arthritis	☐
High blood pressure	☐
Elevated cholesterol	☐
Coronary heart disease	☐
Loss of memory	☐
Reduced cognitive function	☐

More information on essential fatty acids is included in Chapter 3, Chapter 5 and Chapter 8.

Foods rich in essential fatty acids
 ✓ *Fish (especially oily fish such as salmon, trout, mackerel, etc.)*
 ✓ *Nuts and seeds*
 ✓ *Oils*
 ✓ *Enriched eggs.*

7 LIMIT OXIDATIVE DAMAGE TO FATS

Oils rich in polyunsaturated fatty acids such as sunflower or safflower oil are more prone to oxidation (which can go on to cause free radical damage in the body) and this is increased when these oils are heated. Cold vegetable oils provide essential fatty acids and fat-soluble vitamins such as vitamin E and can be included in a healthy anti-ageing diet as salad dressings. In the same way that fats oxidize more readily when they are heated, they also oxidize whenever they are exposed to oxygen (air) and light.

For a healthy salad dressing, choose from rapeseed oil, linseed oil or walnut oil, keep the oils:

▶ *in a dark coloured bottle*
▶ *in a cool place*
▶ *away from direct sunlight*

and add a vitamin E tablet to prevent oxidation!

8 *LIMIT YOUR INTAKE OF FOODS THAT INCREASE FREE RADICAL DAMAGE*

Certain foods contain compounds that will need to be detoxified, which can increase the level of free radical damage in the body. This is because the detoxification process itself can create compounds that are sometimes toxic or carcinogenic. In addition to ensuring that you consume plenty of the nutrients needed for Phase 2 detoxification (see Chapter 4 to remind yourself what these are), the best way to limit free radical damage is to limit the food and drinks that require detoxification.

What to avoid to stay young:
* *Smoking*
* *Drugs*
* *Alcohol*
* *Coffee*
* *Cooked meats*
* *Other 'charcoaled' foods*
* *Food additives such as nitrates and nitrites*
* *Medication wherever possible.*

9 *EAT LESS SUGAR!*

Sugar intake has always been clearly linked with diabetes as it affects the amount of insulin we produce and our pancreatic function. There is also a clear link between diabetes, glaucoma and eye health. More recent research illustrates a link between our intake of sugars or refined carbohydrates (which act like sugars in the body) and insulin resistance and obesity. In turn, these conditions cause increased inflammation and cellular damage in the body, which connects diabetes to an increased risk of coronary heart disease. In addition, research illustrates links between a high intake of sugar or refined carbohydrates and all of the following conditions and diseases:

- *obesity*
- *diverticulosis*
- *cancer*
- *Alzheimer's Disease.*

Insight: Reduce your sugar intake to lower body fat

Although carbohydrates contain fewer calories than fats, consuming too many sugars and refined carbohydrates contributes to weight gain and increases body fat. Any excess carbohydrate, protein or fat can be converted into adipose tissue and stored, and this is more likely to happen when the body is 'flooded' with any of these nutrients. As simple sugars and refined carbohydrates are absorbed into the bloodstream more quickly than starchy carbohydrates such as rice or oats, these sugars are more likely to be converted into fat and stored.

We are also more likely to overeat these types of carbohydrate as the processed foods containing them are made to be very palatable and tasty – they are easy to eat but do not provide much sustenance, so one biscuit is never enough! This means that eating refined carbohydrates usually leads to snacking on similar foods to address flagging blood sugar levels and can lead to conditions such as hypoglycaemia and diabetes. Chapter 7 contains more information on the effect that these foods have on our blood sugar levels.

Protein glycosylation
Protein cross-linking is one of the biological signs of increasing age, and can be caused by having too much glucose in the bloodstream.

Essential protein molecules travel around in our bloodstream, for example:

- ▸ *antibodies*
- ▸ *haemoglobin*
- ▸ *hormones*
- ▸ *enzymes.*

Having too much glucose in the bloodstream can result in glucose molecules 'bumping into' these proteins, and attaching themselves. This damages the proteins and renders them useless. These damaged proteins can reduce skin suppleness and contribute to diseases such as atherosclerosis or Alzheimer's.

Insight: Cut down on sugar to reduce ageing!

Reducing sugars and refined carbohydrates will have several benefits:

1 *You can reduce calorie intake and live longer!*
2 *You won't be affecting your intake of nutrients by cutting out sugars.*
3 *Avoiding cakes, pastries, muffins, biscuits, etc. will also reduce your intake of trans and hydrogenated fats.*
4 *You are less likely to store excess sugar as fat.*

Concentrate on cutting down on cakes, biscuits, ice cream, scones, muffins, sweets, chocolate and white flour products and stop adding sugar to drinks and breakfast cereals. This change alone will reduce the risk of obesity, diabetes, heart disease and some cancers, as well as helping to delay ageing!

10 *LIMIT YOUR ALCOHOL INTAKE AND CHOOSE HEART-HEALTHY RED WINE*

Although a small amount of alcohol may reduce the occurrence of heart disease, consuming any more than one to two drinks daily is detrimental to health.

The detrimental effects of alcohol

- *Alcohol contributes to obesity.*
- *It affects blood sugar metabolism.*
- *It can reduce bone density and increase the risk of osteoporosis.*
- *Heavy consumption of alcohol can cause micronutrient deficiencies through reduced absorption, poor hepatic (liver) storage of nutrients and increased requirements for certain nutrients.*
- *Alcohol consumption has been linked with hypertension and arrhythmias.*
- *It can increase the incidence of gastritis and pancreatic disease.*
- *It causes fatty liver and cirrhosis.*
- *It also contributes to neurological disorders.*
- *It is linked with some cancers, for example, liver cancer.*

Insight: The French paradox

France and other Mediterranean countries have a lower incidence of cardiovascular 'events', despite the same level of risk factors such as diabetes, hypertension and elevated cholesterol levels. It seems that although a similar amount of arterial damage is still caused through atherosclerotic fatty plaques and high blood pressure, this damage is somehow offset through reduced blood clotting in those who consume one to two drinks a day – particularly red wine.

This illustrates the apparent U-shaped relationship between alcohol consumption and heart disease. The reduced clotting decreases the fat laid down in the arteries, which lowers the risk of myocardial infarction, stroke and heart attacks.

Epidemiological data from at least 20 countries in Europe, North America, Asia and Australia shows a 20–40 per cent lower incidence of coronary heart disease amongst those who consume a moderate amount of alcohol, in comparison with non-drinkers or heavy drinkers.

How does it work?

1 *Firstly, ethanol in alcohol and the polyphenols found
predominantly in red wine both exert a relaxing
effect upon the artery walls. This allows the artery to
expand to accommodate higher blood flow or pressure,
preventing damage to the artery wall that might create
atherosclerosis.*

2 *Secondly, drinking one to two alcoholic beverages daily can
increase your 'good' cholesterol (HDL) by approximately
12 per cent. The 'good' cholesterol reduces the amount of
'bad' cholesterol (LDL) in the bloodstream and limits the
risk of atherosclerosis, which is partly caused by this type
of cholesterol when it is oxidized. In addition to this, the
flavonoid anti-oxidants in red wine limit the oxidation of
LDL, further reducing fatty cholesterol deposits.*

3 *Thirdly, red wine polyphenols have an anti-inflammatory
effect and limit clot formation.*

So although alcohol consumption is not specifically recommended,
if you do drink, it seems a good idea to limit consumption to one
to two drinks daily, have a few alcohol-free days each week and
drink red wine as your chosen beverage!

Anti-ageing nutrients

Although each nutrient has its role in the body, there are some
anti-oxidant vitamins and minerals and which have been proven
without doubt to aid longevity and health. These super-nutrients
take pride of place in any anti-ageing diet.

VITAMIN C

Nobel Prize winning scientist Linus Pauling stated that we could live up to 18 years longer by supplementing with vitamin C mega doses. This vitamin has been called the key to longevity, reportedly increasing life span by two to six years, 'reversing the biological clock' by increasing white blood cell count and reducing heart disease by 40 per cent.

Insight: Top tip

Place potatoes, broccoli or cabbage directly into boiling water to limit loss of vitamin C during cooking.

What will vitamin C do for me?
- ✓ *Reduce skin degeneration.*
- ✓ *Reduce gum disease.*
- ✓ *Help to prevent cataracts.*
- ✓ *Reduce the risk of heart disease.*
- ✓ *Reduce the risk of some cancers.*
- ✓ *Support detoxification in the liver.*
- ✓ *Boost collagen formation to maintain a youthful complexion.*
- ✓ *Reduce arterial damage through anti-inflammatory mechanisms.*
- ✓ *Help to reduce LDL or 'bad' cholesterol levels.*
- ✓ *Support immune function.*
- ✓ *Exert anti-inflammatory properties which reduce cellular damage in the skin, liver, kidneys ... in every cell in the body.*

Where to find vitamin C
Citrus fruits, berries, green leafy vegetables, peppers, kiwi fruit.

VITAMIN E

Vitamin E has several cardio-protective benefits, largely due to its anti-oxidant properties that help to prevent cholesterol becoming oxidized and causing atherosclerosis, thrombosis, myocardial infarction, strokes and heart attacks. It has been cited as the most potent anti-oxidant to reduce cholesterol, one study reporting a

40 per cent decrease in cholesterol oxidation after participants took 800 IU of vitamin E daily for three months. Vitamin E supplementation was also shown to reduce heart disease by 41 per cent in a large-scale study over two years.

Vitamin E supplementation offers protection against some cancers through its anti-oxidant, anti-inflammatory and immune-supportive functions.

> ## Insight: Boost your vitamin E content now!
> *By snacking on nuts and seeds.*
> *By drizzling high-quality, cold vegetable oils onto salads.*
> *By adding pine nuts to salads and stir fries.*
> *By adding wheat germ to cereals or yoghurts.*
> *By adding avocado to salad sandwiches, salads and wraps.*

What will vitamin E do for me?
- ✓ *It reduces free radical damage, a significant cause of 'ageing', which is why it's found in so many face and body creams.*
- ✓ *By reducing free radical damage it can reduce the occurrence of 'liver spots' commonly associated with ageing. These are deposits of a pigment called lipofuscin, the residue remaining after the breakdown and absorption of damaged blood cells.*
- ✓ *It supports immune function.*
- ✓ *It can help to alleviate menopausal symptoms.*

Vitamin E works in conjunction with vitamin C, the effects of each vitamin increased by the other, so a healthy diet should be rich in both of these 'anti-ageing' anti-oxidants.

Where to find vitamin E
Vegetable oils, nuts (especially almonds, Brazils and hazelnuts), pine nuts, sunflower seeds, avocado, wheat germ.

BETA CAROTENE

Beta carotene is one of the carotenoids (see Chapter 3 for more information on this group of superfoods).

Heavy cooking can destroy much of the beta carotene in vegetables, but light cooking, mashing or puréeing may enhance its availability and absorption as the plant cell walls are ruptured and open up to release the beta carotene within. It is best absorbed with some fat in the meal, so combine orange fruits with seeds or nuts, and roast pumpkin, sweet potato or carrots with a little olive oil to enhance absorption, providing vitamin E at the same time.

What will beta carotene do for me?

Beta carotene has pro-vitamin A activity, meaning that it can be converted into vitamin A as and when required.

- ✓ *Vitamin A is essential for good visual health.*
- ✓ *It supports immune function.*
- ✓ *It promotes and protects cell differentiation.*
- ✓ *Beta carotene reduces the occurrence of age-related macular degeneration and cataracts.*
- ✓ *It provides protection against heart disease and some cancers.*

Help to reduce skin ageing with beta carotene

Beta carotene has been proven to offer skin protection to sun exposure to the extent that taking beta carotene supplements before sun exposure has been widely recommended. Pack your diet out with beta carotene-rich foods during the summer to enhance skin protection:

Breakfast	Blend cantaloupe melon and peaches with live yoghurt for a super beta carotene smoothie
Lunch	Tortilla wrap with spinach, avocado, peppers, grated carrots, tomatoes, beetroot

(Contd)

| Dinner | Salmon with roasted carrots, sweet potato and squash |
| Snacks | Apricots, mangoes, peaches, nectarines... |

Other carotenoids such as lycopene, found in tomatoes, have also been proven to have similar protective properties. These carotenoids cannot offer complete protection against UV irradiation, but should be included in the diet for a myriad of health benefits, not least their anti-ageing properties.

Where to find beta carotene
Sweet potato, carrots, squash, pumpkin, mango, papaya, apricots, green leafy vegetables.

SELENIUM

As well as being an anti-oxidant, selenium is required for the detoxification process, so it helps to reduce cellular damage in more than one way. It works synergistically with vitamin E, so it's a good idea to consume these two anti-oxidants together. In clinical trials selenium has repeatedly blocked the formation of cancer, and deficiency is common when selenium status has been assessed in cancer patients. Seafood and nuts are excellent sources of selenium.

Where to find selenium
Brazil nuts, sunflower seeds, wholegrain cereals, seafood and offal.

Insight: Natural selenium supplement!
Brazil nuts are rich sources of selenium; eating just one freshly shelled Brazil nut can be as good as taking a selenium supplement!

Nutrition for super skin

Our skin is made up of the compounds and nutrients derived from the food that we eat, so a healthy balanced diet is essential for good skin. In particular, dry, rough, itchy or flaky skin can be symptoms of fatty acid deficiency or imbalance, as these fats help to maintain the structure of our cell membranes. Vitamin E also has an important role in maintaining our cell membranes, and acne, eczema and dry, itchy skin have all been linked with a deficiency of this vitamin.

Wear your food on your face!

For dry skin: mix 5 ml of olive oil with half an avocado and an egg yolk. Apply it to your skin and leave on for 20 minutes before removing with a damp flannel or cotton wool.

Sagging skin as a result of reduced collagen and elastin, wrinkles and other symptoms of ageing are partly due to free radical damage, so a diet rich in anti-oxidants can help to reduce damage to the skin and to the proteins that help to make collagen and elastin. Vitamin A also contributes to skin health – a deficiency of this vitamin causes excess hardening of the skin.

It's no coincidence that skin creams are packed with anti-oxidants such as vitamin A, vitamin C, vitamin E, selenium, Co-Enzyme Q10 or green tea extracts! The question is, can these nutrients actually penetrate the epidermis, or contribute to skin health from the outside? Scientists have differing opinions, but what we do know for sure, is that if these nutrients are included in the diet, they certainly have a positive effect upon our health and our skin.

FOODS FOR SUPER SKIN

All the anti-oxidants previously mentioned will reduce cell damage and improve the appearance of your skin. In particular, adapt your diet as follows for super skin:

- ✓ *Snack on nuts and seeds.*
- ✓ *Add pine nuts and seeds to salads and stir fries.*
- ✓ *Include avocado in wraps, salads and sandwiches.*
- ✓ *Swap meat for salmon or tuna steaks.*
- ✓ *Have peppered mackerel or poached salmon with salads.*
- ✓ *Eat sardines on toast instead of cheese on toast.*
- ✓ *Add linseeds to yoghurts and cereals.*
- ✓ *Use linseed oil as a great salad dressing or add a dash to smoothies.*
- ✓ *Add berries and orange fruits to breakfast cereals.*
- ✓ *Regularly eat brightly coloured fruit salads.*
- ✓ *Eat dark green leafy vegetables and an orange-coloured vegetable for lunch and dinner each day…*
- ✓ *… and don't forget to drink at least eight glasses of water each day!*

A diet for super skin

Breakfast	Fruit salad with mango, papaya, apricots, kiwi and mixed berries, topped with pumpkin seeds and linseeds
Lunch	Salad packed with anti-oxidants – raw peppers, spinach, carrot, beetroot, tomatoes, avocado, olive oil and pine nuts
Dinner	Salmon and sweet potato risotto with wilted spinach
Snacks	Pumpkin seeds, avocado on corn cakes, fruit, raw peppers, carrot and tomatoes

These tips will enhance your intake of all the nutrients needed for healthy skin:

- *vitamin C*
- *vitamin E*
- *beta carotene*
- *selenium*
- *zinc*
- *essential fatty acids.*

Recipe for salmon and sweet potato risotto (serves 2)
2 salmon steaks
1 small onion, sliced
2–3 cloves garlic, finely diced
150 g organic brown rice
2 large handfuls of rocket
Olive oil
2 medium-sized sweet potatoes, roasted

Bake the salmon steaks and roast the sweet potato in olive oil. Meanwhile, cook the risotto as follows: sauté some garlic and onion with a little olive oil. Add the rice, stirring to coat it with the oil/onion/garlic mixture, then add water and allow to simmer (instructions on rice packets will state how much rice per serving and how much water to use). Keep adding water as required until the rice is cooked. Once all the water is absorbed, add the roasted vegetables and baked salmon to the risotto and serve. Spinach or rocket can also be stirred into the risotto just before serving.

SUN DAMAGE

Although we often feel better in ourselves when we have tanned skin, a tan is an indication of sun damage. Photo-ageing damage from the sun includes damage to collagen and elastin, proteins that give skin its strength and elasticity. These proteins decline as we age, allowing skin to become less taut and saggy.

Protective anti-oxidant nutrients such as beta carotene reduce free radical damage by 'quenching' or absorbing free radicals or rogue oxygen molecules which may cause damage to cells. Eating a diet that is rich in anti-oxidants will not only improve your overall health, but will improve the quality of your skin and also help to protect it.

Remember, foods rich in beta carotene include carrots, sweet potato, squash and pumpkins, and fruits such as mangoes, papaya and cantaloupe melon. Some foods contain beta carotene although the orange pigment is hidden, for instance in green leafy vegetables. Other anti-oxidants will also help to reduce skin damage, and including these nutrients in your diet rather than relying on skin creams is likely to be a better skin insurance policy!

Water

Water is vital for efficient metabolism and to help rid the body of toxins and waste products. 70 per cent of our body weight is made up of water; it plumps up the skin, filling the cells and reducing the appearance of wrinkles, and without adequate hydration, our skin can look and feel dry. Adequate water consumption – at least one litre of water daily – is therefore an essential element of good nutrition for healthy skin.

How to increase your water intake
- *Take a filled 1.5 or 2 litre bottle to work or keep it at home with you and drink the water throughout the day – a great way to measure how much you're drinking.*
- *Drink herbal teas or hot water with a slice of lemon or lime as a refreshing alternative to coffee or tea.*
- *Take a small bottle of water with you when you go out in the car or on a walk so you always have something to drink.*
- *It's essential to re-hydrate during and after a workout as you have to replace the water that you have lost as sweat.*
- *Fill up on foods with high water content such as melons, cucumber, tomatoes, pears ...*

Face mask for dehydrated skin

Mix 5 ml of runny honey with a small, ripe, mashed banana and 25 g of oatmeal. Apply it to your skin and leave on for 20 minutes before rinsing off.

Does diet affect your hair and nails?

Both our hair and nails are made from, and affected by, the foods that we eat. Do any of these conditions sound familiar?

▶ *Copper excess can cause hair loss.*
▶ *Copper deficiency can cause hair to be wiry or lack pigmentation.*
▶ *A lack of zinc is illustrated by white specks on nails.*
▶ *Ridged, soft or brittle nails can be a sign of vitamin B deficiency.*
▶ *Poor nails can also indicate a lack of silicon or poor protein intake.*

So, as with the rest of the body, you are what you eat!

NUTRITION FOR HEALTHY HAIR

Dull, lifeless hair can be an indication of fatty acid deficiency, particularly if you also have dandruff and rough or bumpy skin. We cannot form the essential fatty acids in the body, so we have to include them in our diet. There are two fatty acids that are essential – linolenic acid (an omega 3 acid) and linoleic acid (an omega 6 acid). As already mentioned, although most of us have enough omega 6 fats in the diet, we often lack enough omega 3, so fill up on fish or linseeds for a good intake of these essential fatty acids.

Potassium helps to balance the effect of the sodium found in salt and we should consume at least twice as much potassium as sodium. Potassium is concentrated in fruits, vegetables and juices, and most processed foods are rich in sodium, so many of us have an unbalanced intake of these minerals, especially if you also add salt to your food or cooking. Follow these tips to cut back on salt:

▶ *Stop adding salt to cooking – the subtle effect is lost if salt is added to a meal anyway.*

▶ *Stop adding salt to your food on the plate – especially before you've even tasted it!*

▶ *Buy reduced-salt foods and cut back on the use of tinned and packet convenience foods, where much salt is added for taste and to help preserve the food.*

▶ *Cut back on high-salt foods such as cheese, bacon, pizza, crisps, etc.*

NUTRITION FOR GREAT NAILS

Our nails are made up of protein and a combination of minerals, and are dependant upon a healthy, balanced diet for good formation, including a sufficient intake of B vitamins and the essential fatty acids.

Having healthy hair and nails is a product of sufficient protein and a balanced intake of several minerals and vitamins. By eating a healthy balanced diet you should consume enough of all the nutrients required. Follow the Superfood diet in Chapter 3 and you're bound to enjoy shiny hair, super skin and strong nails!

Fiona had always had white specks on her nails and thought it was due to a lack of calcium, even though she ate plenty of dairy foods. She didn't, however, eat meat or shellfish and was unaware that she was lacking zinc in her diet until she had a nutritional consultation. After following the zinc-rich diet and supplement plan prescribed for her, the white specks disappeared as her nails grew and, after a couple of months, the new nail growth finally yielded speck-free nails.

Your anti-ageing guide

FOR BETTER SKIN

▶ *Fill up on foods rich in carotene during the summer months to help protect your skin from the sun: pumpkin, squash, carrots, sweet potato, mango, papaya and green leafy vegetables.*

▶ *Eat foods rich in essential fatty acids to prevent dry skin and pimples, and to reduce inflammatory skin disorders such as eczema or psoriasis.*

▶ *Eat plenty of berries – vitamin C and proanthocyanidins are essential for formation of collagen, a protein in the skin.*

TO REDUCE HEART DISEASE

▶ *Garlic has to be the top cardio-protective food for its anti-clotting, anti-thrombotic and anti-sclerotic properties, as well as its ability to lower cholesterol.*

▶ *Swap meat for fish to reduce saturated fat intake, create healthier cholesterol levels and reduce atherosclerosis.*

▶ *Use cardio-protective olive oil instead of butter or margarine and limit free radical damage by using it in cooking too.*

▶ *Fill up on fruit and vegetables to lower blood pressure, reduce cholesterol levels and limit arterial damage through anti-oxidant content.*

▶ *Eat fibre-rich beans, oats and brown rice to reduce cholesterol.*

▶ *Reduce salt intake to reduce or help avoid hypertension.*
▶ *If you have a tipple, make it a glass of red wine!*

FOR HEALTHY JOINTS AND BONES

▶ *Fill up on bone-building nutrients – calcium, magnesium, zinc, vitamin C, manganese and iron – nuts, seeds, beans and pulses, vegetables and whole grains provide a good source of these nutrients without the drawbacks of eating meat and dairy foods.*
▶ *Limit coffee, alcohol and high protein diets.*
▶ *Eat plenty of berries – vitamin C and proanthocyanidins both support collagen formation and will help to strengthen your joints.*
▶ *Eat anti-inflammatory foods if you have arthritis – fish, linseeds and onions.*
▶ *Give up smoking.*
▶ *Swap dairy milk for soya – the phyto-oestrogen content can help to strengthen bone and reduce osteoporosis.*

TO REDUCE THE RISK OF DIABETES

▶ *Eat high-fibre, whole-grain carbohydrates like brown rice and pulses.*
▶ *Include a little protein in small, regular meals throughout the day: this slows down the absorption of glucose.*
▶ *Follow a low-fat diet and avoid overeating – obesity increases the risk of diabetes.*
▶ *Limit alcohol consumption as this affects blood sugar control.*
▶ *Limit caffeine intake as coffee, tea and fizzy drinks affect glucose control. Choose green tea instead for its catechins which support pancreatic function.*
▶ *Limit salt intake: a poor sodium:potassium ratio is common in diabetes.*

FOR IMPROVED IMMUNE FUNCTION

▶ *Fill up on anti-oxidant rich foods to boost immune function: orange-coloured fruit and vegetables for beta carotene, citrus fruits, berries, kiwi and peppers for vitamin C, nuts, seeds and*

vegetable oils for vitamin E, and whole grains, nuts and seeds for zinc and selenium.
- ▶ Consume foods with anti-inflammatory properties every day – onions, linseeds, fish and garlic.
- ▶ Limit foods that need extra detoxification, such as charcoaled foods.
- ▶ Swap coffee for anti-oxidant rich green tea.

FOR IMPROVED DIGESTION AND BOWEL HEALTH
- ▶ Eat a high-fibre diet with whole grains such as brown rice, beans and pulses, fruit and vegetables making up most of your food consumption.
- ▶ Limit alcohol, coffee, tea, salt, sugar and refined carbohydrates.
- ▶ Limit meat and dairy foods and fill up on inulin-rich vegetables such as asparagus, onion, garlic and chicory for a healthy bowel.
- ▶ Include linseeds for its anti-inflammatory and bowel motility benefits.
- ▶ Drink 1–2 litres of water each day for healthy bowel motility.

FOR IMPROVED MENTAL FUNCTION
- ▶ Eat fish two to four times weekly for the long chain polyunsaturated fats known to benefit cognitive function.
- ▶ Limit stimulants such as coffee, tea, alcohol and sugar – these can cause hyperactivity and behavioural difficulties.
- ▶ Drink anti-oxidant green tea to limit free radical damage to brain cells.
- ▶ Try to eliminate all sources of aluminium in your diet – avoid using aluminium saucepans, foil and medications containing aluminium, for example, indigestion remedies.
- ▶ Eat a zinc-rich diet – fill up on whole grains, pumpkin seeds, seafood and eat lean cuts of meat.

FOR ENHANCED EYE HEALTH
- ▶ Eat orange-coloured fruit and vegetables rich in carotenoids.
- ▶ Fill up on lutein-rich foods such as avocados and green leafy vegetables.

- *Lycopene in tomatoes is another carotenoid that enhances eye function.*
- *Vitamin C-rich berries, kiwi, peppers and citrus fruit will support collagen production and reduce the risk of glaucoma.*
- *Macular degeneration is often linked with arterial disease – follow tips for a healthy heart and your eyes will benefit too!*

THINGS TO REMEMBER

Top ten anti-ageing superfoods:

Oily fish

- ✓ *Enhances memory and cognitive function*
- ✓ *Reduces heart disease*
- ✓ *Enhances skin health*
- ✓ *Reduces inflammatory conditions such as arthritis*

Carotene-rich foods (squash, sweet potato, carrots...

- ✓ *Top nutrient to protect against skin damage*
- ✓ *Anti-oxidant nutrient supporting immune function*
- ✓ *Protects against macular degeneration and cataracts*
- ✓ *Anti-cancer benefits*

Citrus fruits and berries (fruits rich in vitamin C)

- ✓ *Vitamin C provides anti-inflammatory benefits*
- ✓ *Increases white blood cell count and supports immune function*
- ✓ *Prompts beneficial changes in cholesterol ratios, reducing heart disease*
- ✓ *Anti-cancer benefits*

Green tea

- ✓ *Enhances pancreatic function, reducing the risk of diabetes*
- ✓ *Rich in anti-oxidant catechins which fight free radical damage*
- ✓ *Supports immune function*
- ✓ *Anti-carcinogenic properties*

Green leafy vegetables

- ✓ *Proven to protect against heart disease*
- ✓ *Rich in anti-oxidants vitamin C and beta carotene*
- ✓ *Contain nutrients required for detoxification*
- ✓ *Proven to protect against some cancers*

Garlic

- ✓ *Anti-thrombotic, reducing the risk of blood clots and thrombosis*
- ✓ *Anti-bacterial, anti-fungal and anti-microbial, protecting against disease*
- ✓ *Increases 'good' HDL cholesterol and reduces 'bad' LDL cholesterol*
- ✓ *Anti-cancer benefits*

Soya

- ✓ *Contains phytosterols which reduce cholesterol levels*
- ✓ *Has been shown to have anti-cancer properties with some cancers*
- ✓ *Phospholipids in soya enhance liver function*
- ✓ *Phyto-oestrogens in soya can help to reduce menopausal symptoms and counteract osteoporosis*

Foods rich in proanthocyanidins – red grapes, red wine, berries

- ✓ *Rich in anti-oxidant flavonoids to reduce free radical damage*
- ✓ *Reduce inflammation: beneficial for arthritis, skin diseases*
- ✓ *Proven to reduce atherosclerosis and heart disease*
- ✓ *Used in cosmetic preparations to help reduce wrinkling*

Seeds and nuts

- ✓ *Rich in the essential fatty acids for healthy skin, hair and nails*
- ✓ *Linseeds softens the stool, enhancing colon health*
- ✓ *Rich in anti-oxidants vitamin E, zinc and selenium*
- ✓ *Linked with reduced rate of cardiovascular heart disease*

Water

- ✓ *Good hydration helps to prevent dry, wrinkled skin*
- ✓ *Softens the stool, enhancing colon health and toxin elimination*
- ✓ *Supports kidney function and urinary toxin elimination*
- ✓ *As well as being essential for health, it promotes a healthy weight.*

7

Energy boosting foods

In this chapter you will learn:
- *which foods to eat for a quick fix or for sustained energy*
- *how to manage your blood sugar levels*
- *what may be sapping your vitality.*

Having more energy is one of the most common things on our 'better health wish list', yet higher energy levels can be one of the easiest things to rectify through diet. There are a number of foods and nutrients that provide energy, or contribute to the metabolism of energy-yielding nutrients and a good intake of these, in conjunction with reducing any 'energy-robbing' habits, will make a world of difference to your vitality.

Get more energy now!

1 *Drink one to two litres of water daily.*
2 *Cut down on coffee and tea intake.*
3 *Fill up with whole grains – oats, brown rice and beans.*

Fatigue can be due to lack of sleep (or poor quality sleep), stress, a poor diet with either inadequate calorie or nutrient intake, or too many toxins and stimulants. It can also occur as a result of another health condition or disease such as candidiasis (yeast overgrowth), food intolerances, anaemia or chronic fatigue syndrome (ME). Symptoms of these conditions will be addressed later on in this chapter, but it is important to see your doctor for a diagnosis, particularly if your fatigue continues.

For most of us, an inadequate diet or poor lifestyle habits lead to flagging energy levels, so that is where you should begin. Often, in following a better diet, other health conditions that may have been causing fatigue will also improve automatically.

Where do we get energy from?

Although proteins, fats and even alcohol all contain energy, the most important group of foods for energy is the carbohydrates. These foods provide ongoing energy in the form of glucose in our bloodstream and without enough carbohydrate, or glucose, we feel lethargic and tired.

Carbohydrate-rich foods:

- *potatoes*
- *rice*
- *breakfast cereals such as oats or muesli*
- *wholemeal bread*
- *pasta*
- *vegetables*
- *fruit.*

All of these foods contain a mixture of nutrients including some protein and fat, but they contain different types of carbohydrates, known as sugars or starches. A sugar is a simple molecule that is absorbed quickly into the bloodstream. Glucose is one of these sugars and it is glucose that we use for energy. The starches are made up of sugar molecules all joined together to make larger molecules – these take longer to be broken down, digested and absorbed into the bloodstream, so they tend to give us a more sustained release of energy, rather than creating the quick surge of energy that foods high in glucose provide.

Glycaemic Index (GI) and Glycaemic Load (GL)

GLYCAEMIC INDEX (GI)

The Glycaemic Index (GI) is a measure of how quickly the glucose in foods is absorbed into the bloodstream – a low GI will mean the food has low glucose content or contains mostly slow-release starches. A high GI score indicates a food that should give you energy more quickly. Obviously, you can choose to eat certain foods based upon their GI to provide you with a more sustained energy release or a quick burst of energy.

GLYCAEMIC LOAD (GL)

The Glycaemic Load of a food measures the effect that a normal portion of food or drink will have on blood sugar levels. It indicates the type of carbohydrate in a food (the GI) and how much carbohydrate a typical portion contains, and can be calculated as follows:

$$\frac{\text{Glycaemic Index (GI)} \times \text{the weight of available carbohydrate (g)}}{100}$$

The GI and GL of many common foods

FOOD	GI	Carb (g) per portion	GL
Lucozade	95	40	38
White baguette	95	22	21
White rice	87	56	49
Rice cakes	85	6	5
Cornflakes	84	26	22
Gatorade	78	15	12
Watermelon	72	14	10

(Contd)

FOOD	GI	Carb (g) per portion	GL
Mars bar	68	43	29
Digestive biscuits	59	10	6
Banana	55	23	12.5
Baked beans	48	31	15
Orange juice	46	14	6.5
Porridge	42	14	6
Spaghetti	41	49	20
Apple	38	12	4.5
Chick peas	33	24	5
Dried apricots	31	15	4

GI and GL levels

High GI	70 to 100	High GL	20 or more
Medium GI	55 to 70	Medium GL	11 to 19
Low GI	Under 55	Low GL	10 or less

If you check the carbohydrate grams (g) on a food label, the higher the grams per portion, the higher the GL, particularly if a food has a high GI as well, in which case it will give you a quicker release of energy. Although Glycaemic Index indicates whether a food or drink contains a high proportion of glucose in relation to other sugars, not all high GI foods contain large amounts of glucose.

For example, watermelon has a reasonably high GI as most of the sugars are glucose. However, it doesn't have a high Glycaemic Load as so much of it is water; a typical portion contains only 14 g of carbohydrate, in comparison to 40 g in a 250 ml bottle of Lucozade. So if you are looking for something that will give you a quick burst of energy, choose a food or drink with a high GI and a high GL.

Insight: Calculate the GI of your meal

You can add the GI of all the foods in a meal together, and then divide the total by the number of foods eaten to get an average GI figure for the meal, as shown below. This enables you to combine different foods to slow down energy release from high GI foods, or tailor the energy release to suit your requirements. For example,

Baked potato + beans + a yoghurt = 85 + 48 + 33 = 166 divided by 3

This gives an average glycaemic index (GI) of 55 (medium).

Of course, the absorption and digestion time of a food is affected by lots of different factors:

- *Eating fatty or protein foods at the same time as a carbohydrate will slow down the release of glucose.*
- *Eating high-fibre foods also slows down the absorption of glucose.*
- *Combining lower GI or GL foods with high GI/GL foods will reduce the overall GI and GL.*
- *Cooking foods for longer helps to break down the walls of the starch molecules, which makes the energy (glucose) more readily available and will increase the GI.*

Blood sugar control

Many of us live on a blood sugar roller coaster, going from one quick fix to the next, with energy surges following cups of coffee with refined carbohydrate snacks (high GI foods) alternating with energy slumps. Sound familiar?

Although it's a natural mechanism for the body to control blood glucose (blood sugar) levels, it is healthier and more effective to try to create an even keel of energy throughout the day. You can do this by choosing slower release carbohydrates, or eating protein foods at each meal to slow down the release of glucose. Our body naturally produces a hormone called glucagon, which turns the stored energy (glycogen) in our body into glucose. This helps to keep our energy levels fairly stable, and provides energy in between meals. Whenever we consume quick-release carbohydrates which elevate our blood sugar level, we produce a hormone called insulin, which reduces the level of glucose in our bloodstream. It does this in a number of ways:

1 *It increases the amount of glucose that goes into the cells.*
2 *It increases the conversion of glucose into glycogen (its storage form), although we can only store a certain amount (about 90 minutes' worth) of glucose in this way.*
3 *It decreases the use of fat for energy so that we can utilize excess glucose instead.*
4 *It may convert excess glucose into fats.*

Certainly the last two actions of insulin are not conducive to reducing or maintaining body fat levels, and high levels of insulin have been linked to conditions such as obesity, diabetes and heart disease. So although sugary or high GI foods may seem relatively low in calories in comparison to fats, consuming these foods on a regular basis is not a good idea for your waistline or for your health.

There are several problems with constantly using sugary foods or stimulants to provide a quick surge of energy. As discussed, high glucose levels result in insulin release, which reduces the level of glucose in the blood. In some people, this results in low glucose levels again, and a further need for caffeine, sugar or quick release carbohydrates. This can create blood sugar highs and lows throughout the day, increasing your need for sugar and stimulants, which in turn tends to lower your intake of wholesome, nutritious foods. When was the last time you reached for an apple or cup of lentil soup for a quick fix?!

High glucose levels incite insulin release

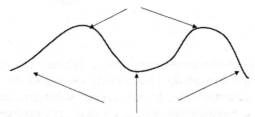

Low blood sugar levels prompt intake of sugar and stimulants.

Figure 7.1 Blood sugar curve.

Janet was missing meals through the day because of work then feeling very drowsy whilst driving home every night. She regularly stopped to buy chocolate to boost her blood sugar levels, but knew this was causing her to gain weight. Simply snacking through the day and having a quick bite to eat before she got in the car after work completely removed the chocolate cravings and kept her awake at the wheel!

Often, when we have the urge to consume something sweet, these foods also contain high levels of fat or calories. Foods such as sweets, biscuits, doughnuts, chocolate and pastries are commonly used to elevate blood sugar levels, providing a high calorie intake with few nutrients. When considering food intake for the day, you are likely to think you have eaten very little as these 'snacks' are not considered as meals and calorie or fat intake is often underestimated, leading to weight gain.

A further problem associated with quick-fix carbohydrates is that they are unlikely to be rich sources of vitamins and minerals, so your diet may be lacking in vital nutrients needed for health and energy. In addition to this, large and frequent fluctuations in blood sugar levels can ultimately result in deficiencies in the nutrients required to manage blood sugar metabolism and once depleted, a lack in these nutrients will affect your ability to manage blood sugar levels properly, potentially leading to hypoglycaemia (low blood sugar) or even diabetes.

Oliver was newly diagnosed with Type 2 diabetes but wanted to try to control it through diet. His current diet of pastries, sweets and quickly absorbed white breads was not helping his blood sugar control, but including protein foods at each meal with slow release carbohydrates quickly provided a steady, controlled level of glucose.

So the best way to manage energy levels is by including slow-release carbohydrates with protein foods in each meal, avoiding blood sugar highs and lows and also reducing your risk of diabetes. Here is an example:

Breakfast	Porridge with yoghurt
Lunch	Mixed bean salad with tuna
Dinner	Salmon risotto with brown rice and vegetables
Snacks	Oat bars, apples and yoghurts

CAN A HIGH PROTEIN DIET HELP BLOOD GLUCOSE CONTROL?

Because of the detrimental effects eating a lot of sugar or refined carbohydrates (those that are processed and have a high GI, such as white bread, doughnuts, etc.) can have on our weight and our health, a number of higher protein diets have been popular over the past few years. Although a high-protein diet is not necessarily a healthy diet, it can help to improve blood sugar and energy levels.

1 *In 'cutting out the carbs', high protein diets have succeeded in reducing our intake of refined and quick-release carbohydrates.*
2 *Protein foods make us feel full, reducing the likelihood of reaching for sugary snacks between meals.*
3 *Eating protein foods with carbohydrates slows down the release of glucose into the bloodstream, reducing the Glycaemic Index of a meal – this can help you to control blood sugar highs and lows.*

However, many high-protein diets are too low in energy-giving carbohydrates and if you are lacking in energy, you may simply need more carbohydrate foods in your diet, particularly if you are currently following a high protein diet.

How much carbohydrate should you eat?

General guidelines recommend that 50 per cent of our calorie intake should come from carbohydrates and that each meal should be based upon a starchy carbohydrate. In addition to that, adding protein foods to each meal will help to slow down glucose absorption. For example:

▶ *Porridge oats with added yoghurt*
▶ *Peppered mackerel with chickpea and mixed bean salad*
▶ *Brown rice with chicken, turkey, fish or tofu.*

Just follow the recommended guidelines by including a starchy carbohydrate in each meal and see how energized you feel.

Insight

For enhanced energy levels and weight management, choose small helpings (approximately 50 g, uncooked for each portion) of whole grain, low GI carbohydrates such as brown rice or oats. Fruit and vegetables tend to contain less carbohydrate but more water, fibre and micronutrients, so these foods are a healthy way of consuming carbohydrates at each meal in addition to the starchy grains and beans.

Energy giving foods

So, taking into account how much carbohydrate a food contains, its Glycaemic Index, and vitamin and mineral levels (as these help to 'unlock' carbohydrate energy for us), what are the best energy giving foods? On the next page there is a list of healthy, nutritious carbohydrates for a quick fix and equally nutritious foods to eat throughout the day to keep energy levels high.

For a quick buzz	To keep you going
Bananas	Porridge
Raisins	Beans on wholemeal toast
Watermelon	Rice and beans, for example, chilli
Watermelon juice	Risotto
Dates	Berry fruit salad with yoghurt
Cereal bar	Nut or seed bar

THE ENERGY YIELDING MICRONUTRIENTS

Along with the energy we find in food, there are a number of micronutrients that are responsible for 'unlocking' or metabolizing this energy. These nutrients naturally occur in carbohydrates, protein and fats to convert food into energy. For example:

▶ *You'll find vitamin B_1 (thiamine) in carbohydrates such as peas, beans and grains such as bread or oats.*
▶ *You'll find vitamin B_2 (riboflavin) in dairy foods, fish and seafood, and vitamin B_3 (niacin) in fish and meat.*

Co-enzyme A

Pantothenic acid is also known as vitamin B_5 and its active form is Co-enzyme A, which is often sold in supplement form specifically marketed to enhance energy levels. This is because it is required to produce energy from carbohydrates, proteins and fats.

Insight: Adrenal support

In nutritional practice, vitamin B_5 is often used to support adrenal function after years of over-stimulation through use of caffeine, smoking and high sugar intake. It is often supplemented in conjunction with vitamin C, as this vitamin is also required for optimal adrenal function. A multi-vitamin, multi-mineral containing vitamin C and vitamin B_5 may help to increase your energy levels, but always improve your diet first!

Vitamin B_5 occurs in many different foods and a healthy, whole food diet should provide ample amounts of this nutrient. However, if your diet relies on many processed foods and you are lacking in energy, or regularly using stimulants such as sugar, coffee or nicotine to lift energy levels, you will benefit from including the following B_5-rich foods in your diet:

- *fresh parsley*
- *broad beans*
- *chicken*
- *trout*
- *mushrooms*
- *avocado*
- *tahini (sesame seed paste).*

Although the specific foods listed are rich sources of these vitamins, the B vitamins usually occur together in a wide range of foods, and this is the best way of ensuring that you consume enough. In processed foods there is a high loss of vitamins, so much so that many foods are fortified with them (check out the front of your cereal packet!), but it's always best to obtain these nutrients from the foods that they naturally occur in. In eating a wide range of foods you will also consume the minerals that can affect energy levels, such as iron, magnesium and zinc.

Water

Although water contains no calories – and therefore no actual energy – it has a major effect upon our energy levels and performance. This is because it is fundamental to energy metabolism in the body. Dehydration causes several symptoms, many of which are indications of a lack in energy! How many of these symptoms sound familiar? Tick them off now, and then check the list again after you've increased your water intake to see if you have improved.

▶ *Lethargy* ☐
▶ *Lack of focus* ☐
▶ *Reduced attention span* ☐
▶ *Mind feeling 'foggy'* ☐
▶ *Sluggishness* ☐
▶ *Fatigue* ☐
▶ *Headaches* ☐
▶ *Feeling light-headed* ☐
▶ *Lack of energy!* ☐

Score before increased water intake ☐

Score after drinking eight glasses of
water for two consecutive days ☐

Many of us are in a state of chronic dehydration, meaning that we are not consuming enough fluid to work at an optimal level. You should be consuming between one and two litres of water daily, which equates to approximately eight large glasses of water, and be producing urine that is plentiful and a very pale straw colour!

Insight

Quite simply, dehydration could easily be the reason for a lack of energy, and drinking more water may be all you need to do to increase vitality!

HOW TO INCREASE YOUR FLUID INTAKE

Remember the following tips from Chapter 6? Drinking more water will enhance overall health and vitality as well as contributing to great-looking skin, and can even help with weight loss.

▶ *Fill a large bottle of water up each morning and drink it throughout the day. You'll be surprised how keeping the bottle* on your desk at work, or on the table at home, can prompt you to keep taking sips. Drinking water from the bottle makes it easy to measure your fluid intake as well.

▶ On colder days drink hot water with a slice of refreshing lemon or lime, or try herbal teas. These hot drinks contribute more to fluid levels than tea or coffee as tea and coffee are diuretics and cause us to lose water (also, see the next paragraph on caffeinated drinks and energy levels).

▶ Make sure you always have a water bottle with you when you exercise as you need to replace lost fluid with extra water. Weigh yourself before and after your exercise session – whatever weight you've lost is water and needs replacing! Drink a pint of water for each pound lost in weight. For high-intensity activities, or in hot weather, drink a little more.

▶ Make water more interesting by adding ice and a slice of lemon or lime to a nice wine glass.

▶ Fluid also comes from the foods we eat, so fill up on soups and stews in winter, and fruits and salad vegetables with a high fluid content in summer, such as cucumber, tomatoes, pears or watermelon.

Insight: Measure your fluid intake

Keep a note of your water intake in a food diary similar to that in Chapter 2, or note down each glass of water in your diary or on a note pad. A good tip is to drink a glass of water for each cup of coffee or tea you have – this boosts your fluid intake and helps to offset the diuretic effect that these drinks have. If you drink your water beforehand you might find you don't need your regular brew after all!

Caffeinated drinks

Coffee and tea affect both our fluid and energy levels. Due to some of the compounds these products contain, they have a diuretic effect – in other words, they stimulate the production of urine and loss of fluid from the body. Although you may be consuming plenty of fluid in your mugs of tea or coffee, you are also prompting fluid loss and often taking essential minerals such as potassium and magnesium along with it.

Insight: Did you know?

When we consume caffeinated products, our adrenal glands are stimulated to produce adrenaline. Adrenaline is our 'fight or flight' hormone and mobilizes stored energy (carbohydrates and fats), creating an increase in glucose in the bloodstream. This is what creates the energy surge that you experience when you have a cup of tea or coffee, or a glass of caffeinated cola.

On a positive note, a moderate amount of caffeine has been shown to improve focus, memory and immediate energy levels, but if we use caffeine as a constant pick-me-up, we risk becoming attuned to it and needing larger amounts. We often use caffeine to improve our energy levels, but it can, if used too frequently, also result in energy slumps in between 'fixes'.

Regular consumption of coffee (more than two to three cups daily) can result in the same blood sugar highs and lows you would experience with a regular intake of high GI or sugary foods. Once blood glucose levels are elevated after coffee consumption, insulin is released to reduce the high level of glucose; repeated, high levels of glucose in the bloodstream can lead to difficulties in blood glucose regulation, insulin resistance and hyperinsulinaemia (too much insulin in the bloodstream), hyperglycaemia (too much glucose in the bloodstream), diabetes, obesity and denatured protein molecules known as protein glycosylation (see Chapter 6 for more information on this).

So the habitual coffee and Danish/biscuit/muffin pick-me-up may be a short-term solution to flagging energy, but it isn't the ideal way to create healthy, sustained energy levels.

Stress

In the same way that caffeine stimulates our adrenal glands to produce adrenaline, stress has the same effect. Following the 'stressed' message from the brain, our adrenal glands produce adrenaline, which results in the conversion of glycogen (stored energy) into glucose. Of course, in today's lifestyle, we are rarely in a 'fight or flight' situation when adrenaline is produced and simply do not need this extra energy circulating in our bloodstream. Adrenaline also causes fatty acids to be mobilized from stored adipose tissue, which is a good thing if these fats are going to be used for energy, but think what you were doing when you last felt stressed or drank a cup of coffee (which creates a similar reaction to stress). The chances are that you were not using too much energy up. Were you sat at your desk at work? Worrying about something at home? Sat in a traffic jam?

When the mobilized fats (and extra glucose) are not used up as energy, they will eventually be stored again. However, with repeated, regular adrenaline release, chronic health conditions can begin to form. As well as the increased glucose in the bloodstream contributing to protein glycosylation damage and insulin resistance, evidence suggests that circulating fatty acids contribute to atherosclerosis, the fatty plaques on the inside of arteries, linking stress (or simply adrenaline release) to an increased risk of heart disease. So if you are riding a daily roller coaster of energy highs and lows, it is likely that your adrenal function could do with a little support!

Adrenal superfoods

The adrenal glands play a large part in regulating our blood sugar levels and repeated stress, or a high intake of caffeine or sugary foods can tax adrenal function. There are some nutrients which are used regularly by the adrenal glands and an ample supply is required for adrenal health and optimal function. Any diet aimed at improving vitality should include foods rich in vitamin C and the B vitamins, especially vitamin B_5, pantothenic acid.

Foods rich in vitamin C	Foods rich in B vitamins
Citrus fruits	Brown rice
Berries	Wholemeal bread
Broccoli	Dairy foods
Peppers	Meat and fish
Green leafy vegetables	Beans and pulses

For an energy boost – serves 2

100 g fresh blackberries
150 ml fresh orange juice
1 inch piece fresh ginger, finely grated
1 medium pear
Blitz all the ingredients in a blender until smooth. Drink immediately!

Health conditions that can sap vitality

FOOD ALLERGIES

If something obvious such as stress, lack of sleep or not enough water or carbohydrate foods in your diet is not to blame for flagging energy levels, then food sensitivity, food intolerance or food allergy are amongst the most likely culprits, along with candidiasis. Many allergens (the substances responsible for causing a reaction) are eaten frequently and are often favourite foods; this can result in chronic, sometimes debilitating effects upon health, and because of the frequent assault on our immune system and detrimental effects within the body, a food allergy can significantly reduce vitality.

We often crave foods that we are sensitive or even allergic to! Make a list of the foods or drinks that you crave; foods/drinks you look forward to having; foods/drinks that make you feel good immediately after consuming them; and foods and drinks that you consume every day. If you have an intolerance to anything, it's likely to be on your list!

Whilst an allergy would produce allergens in the blood (this is what skin and blood tests are looking for in food allergy tests), a sensitivity or intolerance does not create an immunological reaction that could be measured by antibodies, but there is little other difference between sensitivity or intolerance and allergy to a food or drink. Hence, the term food allergy is commonly used to refer to all three conditions, and the term 'allergen' is used to refer to the offending food or drink.

These are symptoms that often accompany food allergies. If you can tick two or more, it may be worth considering an intolerance to something you regularly eat or drink:

▶ *Fatigue* ☐
  (sometimes immediately after eating a specific food, sometimes chronic fatigue, which may even be momentarily 'improved' by the 'allergen')
▶ *Excess gas, flatulence, heartburn or stomach/bowel* ☐
  cramps
▶ *Diarrhoea, constipation and poor bowel movements* ☐
▶ *Cravings for the 'allergen'* ☐
▶ *Blood sugar fluctuations* ☐
▶ *Atopic conditions (asthma, eczema, hay fever)* ☐
▶ *Inflammatory conditions such as rheumatoid arthritis,* ☐
  irritable bowel syndrome, ulcerative colitis, etc.
▶ *Moodiness, inability to concentrate, hyperactivity and* ☐
  depression

Whilst this list is not exhaustive, it includes many of the most common symptoms associated with a food allergy.

Fixed, variable, cyclic and masked food allergies

FIXED

You will probably know if you have a fixed food allergy as
the reaction occurs immediately after consumption and is often
acute.

VARIABLE

A variable allergy may not occur each time the food or liquid is
consumed, and may only happen if eaten with other specific foods,
or in conjunction with certain medications.

CYCLIC

This is quite a common type of food allergy – although the
reaction occurs each time the allergen is consumed, this may
only happen when the suspect food is consumed regularly. It is
worth remembering that many food allergies do not produce
acute reactions, and it is very common to be unaware of symptoms
or fail to link symptoms to eating certain foods. However, the list
of common symptoms above may include conditions that
you regularly suffer from and you may be able to make a link
between your symptom(s) and eating a particular food. Many
people find that they have an adverse reaction to wheat products
such as bread, yet after a period of exclusion from the diet, they
find they can eat small amounts infrequently without apparent
effect. However, if the frequency of consumption is increased
again, the symptoms of intolerance return. This phenomenon has
resulted in the rotation diet, where foods of the same 'food family'
are not consumed any more regularly than once every five days
after a period of complete exclusion which would normally last at
least three weeks.

MASKED

Consumption of a food or drink to which we have a masked allergy may not seem to cause any untoward symptoms. In fact, you may even feel initially better for having consumed it and, because of this, will probably crave the masked allergen. Common culprits are bread, chocolate, coffee and citrus fruits. However, once the initial feeling of improved well-being has worn off, you are left with the common symptoms of food allergy, often including exhaustion and fatigue.

Case study

Jeanette had struggled with flagging energy levels and weight gain for years and tried every 'diet' she came across with no long-term success. She finally consulted a nutritional therapist who suggested cutting out wheat, eggs and dairy to see how she felt. As soon as she stopped eating wheat Jeanette felt so much better, had an amazing amount of energy and began to lose weight, even though the bread had been replaced by rice and beans, and her calorie intake had not been reduced that much. She can now tolerate a little wheat in her diet with no adverse effects, but lethargy returns as soon as she increases her wheat intake to more than once or twice a week.

It is common to be allergic or sensitive to more than one food at a time and for this to be a long-term problem that evades diagnosis. It is also common to have more than one type of food allergy, cyclic and masked, for example. A food allergy may be present from birth, or it may suddenly occur during adult life. Food sensitivity or intolerance often develops over time, with initial reactions to a food ignored, and the increased frequency of a specific allergen creating an 'adaptive' phase during which you may initially feel better for consuming it, and therefore unwittingly eat it more frequently. Finally, consuming the food or drink in question will no longer provide the 'quick fix' and temporary feeling of well-being, and you are left with the chronic fatigue and other symptoms that a food allergy or sensitivity can cause.

Insight: The most common food allergies

▶ *Dairy foods including milk, cream, yoghurt and cheese (particularly cow's milk and cow's milk products)*

▶ *Wheat products, for example, bread and pasta*

▶ *Gluten (a type of protein found in cereals such as wheat, rye and oats)*

▶ *Eggs*

▶ *Citrus fruits, for example, oranges or grapefruits*

▶ *Coffee*

▶ *Chocolate.*

Additional information regarding common allergens

▶ *Although dairy foods are a common allergen, some people can still tolerate products made from sheep or goats' milk.*

▶ *Peanuts and shellfish are well known for causing immediate and acute allergic reactions of a different nature to that linked with lack of energy.*

▶ *Coeliac disease is a permanent allergy to wheat gluten with genetic and autoimmune traits, as the immune system, in reacting to gluten, also attacks cells within the small intestine, resulting in poor absorption of several nutrients that would normally be absorbed in the small intestine. The gluten found in oats, barley and other cereals may or may not be tolerated in coeliacs.*

What to do if you think you may have a food allergy

1 *You can try to eliminate key allergens from your diet, but this is best done with the help of a qualified practitioner as they will exclude all traces of allergens (it is often difficult to remove all traces of common allergens as substances such as dairy, eggs and wheat are often added to processed foods). A qualified practitioner will also ensure that the exclusion diet is healthy and balanced, with no nutrients lacking.*

2 *If you suspect you may be allergic or sensitive to one of the common allergens, you can try to exclude it from your diet and keep a food diary of how you feel, whether you experience any symptoms, etc. Ideally, an allergen should be excluded for three weeks to allow all traces to be removed from the body, although you may notice a difference in energy levels and other symptoms immediately, or within a few days.*

3　By re-introducing the suspected allergen back into the diet and noting energy levels and any other symptoms, you may be able to identify a food sensitivity or allergy. You then need to decide whether you want to continue eating that food, with the resulting symptoms, or exclude it from the diet. It is best to consult a nutritionist before excluding any major food or food group from the diet to avoid creating nutrient deficiencies. If you are breastfeeding, pregnant or taking any medication, you should also consult with your doctor before making any dietary adjustments.

4　When trying to identify a food allergen, you can exclude more than one suspect food simultaneously, but must re-introduce each food individually otherwise it is impossible to know which food is responsible for causing your symptoms. Remember that it is quite common to be sensitive or allergic to more than one food.

CANDIDIASIS

Candida albicans is a yeast organism that naturally lives in our gut and bowel. However, poor bowel conditions create exactly the right environment for our 'good' bacteria to die off and for organisms like Candida to grow. Candidiasis can manifest as thrush, athlete's foot, or yeast infections in the nails, mouth or stomach. Lifestyle habits that can lead to a poor bowel environment that will encourage Candida overgrowth include the following – tick them off to see if you have a lifestyle that may be encouraging Candida overgrowth!

▶ *Lots of sugar and refined carbohydrates such as white* ☐
   bread
   (Candida feeds on sugar, so eating any type of food that increases glucose levels will feed a Candida overgrowth.)

▶ *Long-term use of the contraceptive pill or HRT* ☐
   (These medications have been linked with higher incidences of thrush.)

▶ *Courses of antibiotics* ☐

▶ *Long-term use of corticosteroid medication for* ☐
   rheumatoid arthritis, asthma or eczema
   (These drugs can depress immune function, making it easier for the Candida organism to grow.)

- ▶ *Regular use of non-steroidal anti-inflammatory medication*
  (These tablets can irritate the gut lining, increasing the likelihood of a 'leaky gut' as the gut membrane becomes more porous.) ☐
- ▶ *Alcohol consumption* ☐
  (This increases thrush as it acts in a similar way to sugar in the body.) ☐
- ▶ *High intake of meat and dairy produce* ☐
  (This creates poor conditions for the 'good' bacteria in our bowel, but an ideal environment for other organisms such as Candida.)
- ▶ *Repeated stress* ☐
  (Stress has an acute effect upon the gut – anyone with irritable bowel syndrome will attest to that! It can cause decreased acid production in the stomach, leading to a more alkaline environment in which yeast will thrive. Stress also suppresses immune function, making it less likely that our body will fight a Candida overgrowth.)

Insight: Did you know?

Antibiotics kill our 'good' bacteria as well as the 'bad' bacteria, creating the ideal opportunity for Candida to thrive once our 'good' bacteria are reduced. Many women commonly experience thrush after taking antibiotics, so much so that some doctors will advise taking a probiotic when prescribing antibiotics.

Anything that limits the growth of healthy bacteria in the bowel will produce favourable conditions for 'bad' bacteria and fungal organisms such as Candida albicans to thrive. This imbalance in our internal flora is known as dysbiosis.

There are many symptoms that might indicate Candida overgrowth, most notably a yeast infection such as thrush or athlete's foot. Fatigue is just one of the symptoms that might accompany these conditions, though candidiasis can be present without an obvious yeast infection. Now you've considered your lifestyle to see if you may be encouraging a Candida overgrowth which may be affecting your energy levels – here is a list of common symptoms that occur when candidiasis is present. If several of these symptoms sound familiar, you may well be experiencing gut dysbiosis and/or candidiasis, which could be sapping your energy levels.

Common symptoms of candidiasis

- ▶ *Recurring cystitis* ☐
- ▶ *PMS and/or endometriosis* ☐
- ▶ *Allergies to food or asthma/eczema* ☐
- ▶ *Food cravings, especially for sugar, bread, chocolate or alcohol* ☐
- ▶ *Hypoglycaemia or an inability to control blood sugar levels* ☐
- ▶ *Abdominal bloating, flatulence, heartburn and indigestion* ☐
- ▶ *Poor bowel motility, diarrhoea or constipation, itchy rectum* ☐
- ▶ *Fuzzy head, inability to focus, poor concentration* ☐
- ▶ *Mood swings and depression* ☐

What to do if you think you may have dysbiosis/candidiasis

1 *Cut out sugars, alcohol and refined carbohydrates from your diet.*
2 *Limit your consumption of meat and dairy foods and increase your intake of vegetables and brown rice. In particular, eat garlic and onion daily with asparagus, Jerusalem artichoke or chicory as these foods have anti-fungal properties and will promote the growth of 'good' bacteria in the bowel.*

(Contd)

3 Limit fruit, dried fruit and fruit juice intake – although these foods are healthy, they are still a concentrated source of sugar.
4 Omit fermented products such as vinegar from your diet for the time being, and try to avoid foods which may harbour yeast organisms such as shelled nuts. If you do eat nuts, choose unshelled. Mushrooms are best omitted as they are a fungi and may encourage fungal growth.
5 Try to avoid using the medications listed earlier.
6 Invest in a good probiotic supplement containing Lactobacillus and Bifidobacterium species.

If fatigue or any other symptoms persist, see your doctor for a diagnosis and consult a registered nutritionist who will be able to provide an anti-Candida diet which also boosts immune function and enables you to re-build a healthy bowel flora.

ANAEMIA

There are several types of anaemia, but one of the most well-known forms is iron deficiency anaemia, which results from either low iron content in the diet, or an inability to absorb iron effectively. This causes a reduction in oxygenated haemoglobin in the blood, therefore affecting energy production and leading to fatigue. Iron does have other uses in the body, and as well as fatigue, symptoms of iron deficiency can include insomnia, lack of appetite, a sore tongue, or gastritis and bowel complaints.

Iron-rich foods:
▶ *Meats*
▶ *Offal*
▶ *Seafood*
▶ *Eggs.*

A vegetarian or vegan diet is most likely to create iron deficiency.
Green leafy vegetables do contain excellent levels of iron, but
the ferric form of iron from plant sources is best absorbed in the
presence of vitamin C, as this alters the iron molecule to a form
more easily absorbed in the gut. As usual, nature already provides
this in unprocessed foods, combining iron with vitamin C in green
leafy vegetables, for example.

Boosting iron intake for vegetarians

For a vegetarian iron-rich meal or snack, combine
foods rich in iron with those rich in vitamin C. Make
your own energy-boosting combinations from the lists
below:

Vegetarian iron-rich foods	Vitamin C-rich foods
Pine nuts	Berries and blackcurrants
Cashew nuts	Citrus fruits
Oats or enriched breakfast cereals	Orange or cranberry juice
Dried apricots and loganberries	Green leafy vegetables
Fenugreek and fennel seeds	Broccoli
Lentils and peas	Peppers

Because of menstruation the iron requirement for females is higher
than that for men. For women aged 19 to 50, the Reference
Nutrient Intake (recommended daily amount) is 14.8 mg/day,
whereas for men it is 8.7 mg/day.

Symptoms of anaemia include the following:

▶ *a pale complexion*
▶ *lack of colour in the mucous membranes underneath the eyelids*
▶ *breathlessness upon exertion*
▶ *listlessness and fatigue.*

Other forms of anaemia include pernicious anaemia, resulting from a lack of vitamin B_{12}, aplastic anaemia, where the formation of red blood cells is affected, and also genetic forms of anaemia such as sickle cell anaemia. If plenty of iron-rich foods are included in your diet yet fatigue prevails, you should visit your doctor, as a blood test can confirm whether any type or level of anaemia is present.

INSOMNIA

Lack of sleep is clearly detrimental to energy levels, but whilst you may have made this obvious connection, you might not realize how much your diet can affect your sleep pattern. Second to stress, our brain is most affected by the availability or excess of nutrients from our diet, creating a cycle of poor sleep, reduced energy levels and use of stimulants, as shown below.

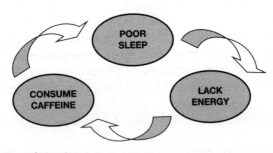

Figure 7.2 *Caffeine and insomnia.*

Is caffeine causing your insomnia?

Consumption of caffeinated drinks is an obvious cause of insomnia. Some people are more susceptible to the effects of caffeine, so you may need to make the following adjustments to your diet if you think this affects you:

▶ *Stop drinking coffee and tea after lunchtime.*
▶ *Avoid caffeine altogether.*
▶ *Limit or avoid other drinks and foods such as green tea, fizzy drinks and chocolate as these also contain caffeine.*

Alcohol also disrupts our sleep, so this should also be eliminated from the diet if you have trouble sleeping.

Another possible cause of insomnia is iron deficiency, so by making sure you have enough iron-rich foods in your diet, you may inadvertently 'cure' both fatigue and insomnia! Too much copper in the diet heightens brain activity which can make it difficult to 'switch off' and get to sleep, yet certain foods actually enhance relaxation and induce sleep. Try these supper recipes for a good night's sleep – it may be all you need to revamp your energy levels!

Sleepy supper recipes

Mix porridge oats with soya milk and add a pinch of cinnamon. Add a spoon of goat or sheep milk yoghurt, raspberries and flaked almonds.

Mix sliced avocado and boiled new potatoes with spinach leaves and alfalfa then add strips of turkey breast.

CHRONIC FATIGUE SYNDROME (ME)

Along with extreme, chronic fatigue, other symptoms of chronic fatigue syndrome may include any of the following:

▶ *tender muscles, joints or lymph nodes*
▶ *poor sleep*

- *forgetfulness*
- *anxiety*
- *depression*
- *headaches.*

However, any of these symptoms would be combined with an inability to function properly over a period of at least six months. Careful medical diagnosis is essential as the symptoms are so varied and many of them may be caused by disorders other than ME.

This is difficult to diagnose and to treat – either with orthodox medication or through naturopathic or dietary means. However, improving general eating habits and following dietary guidelines for specific symptoms such as insomnia will certainly be beneficial and, as an aspect of immune deficiency is involved, following a diet rich in anti-oxidants may also help to boost immune function. Some nutritional therapists specialize in helping people with ME and most nutritionists will be able to provide good dietary advice that may help. Contact the British Association for Nutritional Therapy or the Nutritional Therapy Council for registered practitioners in your area.

THINGS TO REMEMBER

Many things can cause poor energy levels, but by eating a healthy diet you are likely to boost vitality and improve your health at the same time. By improving your diet, you may also find that health conditions which normally sap vitality are largely improved. These are all simple things to do – try to do most of them for most of the time and you're bound to notice a difference!

✓ *Drink at least eight large glasses of water daily.*

✓ *Reduce your caffeine intake (tea and coffee).*

✓ *Limit alcohol intake.*

✓ *Limit sugary and high GI processed foods in the diet (for example, biscuits).*

✓ *Include slow-release (low GI) starchy carbohydrates in each meal to provide sustained energy until your next meal.*

✓ *Add a nourishing protein food to each meal to help slow down energy release from carbohydrate foods.*

✓ *Eat regularly throughout the day to provide sustained energy and avoid blood glucose lows.*

✓ *Only use healthy high GI quick-release carbohydrates when you need an energy boost (bananas, raisins, watermelon).*

✓ *Eat a diverse range of food – a varied diet is more likely to provide you with all the minerals and vitamins you need for health – and energy!*

8

Food for thought

In this chapter you will learn:
- *which foods affect our mood*
- *all about fish oil supplements*
- *tips to boost brain power.*

Although it is easy to understand how what we eat can affect our energy levels or cause weight gain, it may be more difficult to make connections between what we eat and how we think and feel, yet they are intrinsically linked. For example, we need a constant source of glucose (from carbohydrates) for our brain to work – when our blood glucose levels drop we begin to lose concentration and focus, we become moody and stressed, and immediately feel better once we have eaten. Groundbreaking research has repeatedly shown links between fatty acid deficiency and impaired cognitive function, with conditions such as dementia, attention deficit hyperactivity disorder, depression, anxiety, dyslexia and other mental health conditions often responding well to fatty acid supplementation and an improved diet. There are also many micronutrients that affect the functioning of the brain and important links have been made between food and mood and several mental health conditions.

Boost brain power now!

- ▶ *Eat regularly to maintain a constant source of energy for the brain.*
- ▶ *Eat fish at least twice weekly – the long chain fatty acids are needed for mental function.*
- ▶ *Snack on zinc-rich pumpkin seeds – this mineral is vital for good mental function.*

Let's begin by finding out what makes us feel good.

Serotonin

Serotonin is a neurotransmitter enabling chemical messages to travel in our brain; it is also known as the feel-good hormone. Serotonin is formed from an essential amino acid called tryptophan.

Tryptophan-rich foods:

- ✓ *turkey*
- ✓ *chicken*
- ✓ *avocados*
- ✓ *bananas*
- ✓ *broccoli*
- ✓ *spinach.*

As well as eating foods rich in tryptophan, eating carbohydrate foods can also boost serotonin formation. The insulin released when we eat carbohydrate foods such as rice, oats or potatoes indirectly increases the amount of tryptophan taken up by the brain cells. More tryptophan leads to more serotonin, which boosts our mood and helps us to relax. Serotonin also initiates sleep.

Chocolate – friend or foe?

Chocolate is one of the foods most commonly used to lift our mood; chocolate craving has been included as a symptom for medical conditions such as pre-menstrual syndrome and seasonal affective disorder. Chocolate is said to be an aphrodisiac and in the eighteenth century it was used as a medicine! There's no doubt that eating chocolate can make us feel better, but is this psychological or physiological? Can chocolate really be good for us?

HOW DOES CHOCOLATE LIFT THE MOOD?

There are several ingredients in chocolate that contribute to craving, mild addiction and mood improvement.

1 *Firstly, the sugar and caffeine in chocolate elevates our blood sugar levels, the sugar being absorbed into our bloodstream as glucose, and the caffeine stimulating the conversion of stored carbohydrate (glycogen) into glucose, elevating our blood glucose levels further.*
2 *Secondly, the elevated glucose levels stimulate insulin production, this in turn increases the amount of available tryptophan taken up by brain cells and converted into serotonin, the feel-good hormone.*
3 *Thirdly, chocolate also contains a variety of other compounds including theobromine, which acts alongside caffeine as*

*a stimulant, anandamides that have a subtle cannabis-
like effect on the brain, and a number of amines including
phenylethylamine, which is produced naturally in the brain
and released at times of emotional arousal.*

Insight: The best chocolate fix

In one study, white chocolate had no effect upon cognitive
function, but dark and milk chocolate both exhibited
psychopharmacological activity (ability to affect mental
function). These effects are due to the combination of
stimulants caffeine and theobromine. A small bar of dark
chocolate can contain more caffeine than a cup of instant
coffee, useful as a pick-me-up but maybe not a good idea just
before bedtime!

No wonder chocolate lifts our mood!

The best type of chocolate

Chocolate	Properties
Dark	▶ A higher percentage of cocoa solids – no less than 35 per cent ▶ Less added sugar, giving it a more bitter taste but making it a slightly healthier option ▶ The higher the percentage of cocoa solids in the chocolate, the richer the taste and higher the level of anti-oxidants ▶ Plain chocolate also contains iron and magnesium, both nutrients that have been proven to lift mood, especially when deficiencies in these minerals are present

(Contd)

Milk	▶ Milk chocolate generally has the same constituents as plain chocolate but with added milk
	▶ Comparing two bars of chocolate of the same size, the added milk dilutes and reduces the amount of added cocoa solids
White	▶ White chocolate contains cocoa butter, vanilla and lots of added sugar, making it the least healthy type of chocolate

Do you have monthly chocolate cravings?
Magnesium levels can be low during the pre-menstrual period, which may be a reason for the common 'chocolate cravings' experienced at this time of the month. Trials have shown significantly improved mood changes in women taking magnesium supplements. Iron status is likely to be low during and immediately after menstruation, causing an increased requirement and potential craving for foods rich in this mineral, such as red meat, seafood or eggs.

So if you suffer with PMT, filling up on magnesium-rich foods may help – try eating more of these throughout the month, and remember, it may take a number of months to increase your magnesium levels before you notice a difference.

Magnesium-rich foods:

✓ *cauliflower*
✓ *bananas*
✓ *pumpkin*
✓ *brown rice*
✓ *nuts and seeds*
✓ *and, of course, maybe a little dark chocolate!*

Check out the difference in mineral content between 100 g of milk, white and dark chocolate the table opposite.

Mineral content in chocolate

	White	Milk	Plain
Magnesium	26	50	89
Iron	0.2	1.4	2.3
Zinc	0.9	1.1	1.3
Manganese	0.02	0.22	0.63

(Figures are shown in mg/100 g. Taken from McCance and Widdowson's
The Composition of Foods, 6th Ed.)

Insight: Can chocolate be good for mind and body?

Dark chocolate has even been heralded by some as a
'superfood' due to its anti-oxidant content. One study found
higher levels of anti-oxidant flavonoids in dark chocolate
than in red wine and green tea; also separate studies on cocoa
(the active ingredient of chocolate) have illustrated a blood
pressure-lowering effect.

So it's not all bad news for chocolate, but if you're going to indulge
(because it does contain a significant amount of calories, sugar
and fat, don't forget!), use it as an occasional treat and it will do
more to lift your mood than if you ate it every day – as with all
stimulants. Choose dark chocolate to benefit from the extra anti-
oxidants and minerals and maybe a little of what you fancy really
will do you good!

Brain food – fish and fish oils

'Fish makes you brainy' is an old wives' tale, but is there any truth in
it? Existing evidence indicates that many individuals would benefit
from eating more omega 3 fatty acids – the type of fatty acids found

in fish. Research has repeatedly shown improvements in memory and cognitive performance following consumption of fish or fish oil supplements, and evidence suggests that a deficiency of, or imbalance in certain polyunsaturated fatty acids may contribute to conditions such as dyslexia, autism and attention deficit hyperactivity disorder. Higher consumption of seafood across entire nations has been linked with protection against depression, bipolar disorder and seasonal affective disorder, and there are significant correlations between worldwide fish consumption and rates of depression.

How does it work?

▶ *The brain contains a high proportion of fatty tissue, of which 65 per cent is eicosapentanoic acid (EPA) and docosahexanoic acid (DHA) – these are the long chain fatty acids found in fish.*
▶ *DHA is found in the structure of the brain, whereas EPA improves blood flow to the brain, also boosting brain function and acting as a natural anti-inflammatory. These fatty acids are essential for normal brain development and function.*
▶ *They form part of the nerve sheath that surrounds the nerve cells, maintaining membrane flexibility and providing essential insulation for electrical messages and signals to pass from one nerve cell to another, creating our thought processes.*

Insight
Remember, tinned fish loses much of its natural oil during the canning process, so tinned fish such as tuna will only contain approximately the same amount of omega 3 oils as fresh white fish.

What if I don't eat fish?

▶ *You could take a fish oil supplement.*
▶ *You could eat plenty of nuts and seeds, especially linseeds and linseed oil, which contain fats that can be converted into these longer chain fatty acids in the body.*

- *Olive oil is not particularly rich in omega 3 fats, but contains considerably less omega 6 fats than most other oils.*
- *Rapeseed oil is a rich source of omega 3 fats and also has less than half the amount of omega 6 fats found in other vegetable oils such as sunflower oil.*
- *Linseed oil contains an even lower proportion of omega 6 fats and has the highest amount of omega 3 oils available in a vegetable oil.*

Good sources of omega 3 fats	Fish-free options
Sardines	Linseeds or linseed oil
Salmon	Walnuts
Trout	Pumpkin seeds
Herring	Omega 3 fortified eggs
Pilchards	Green leafy vegetables

The fats found in the non-fish sources listed above are not rich in EPA or DHA, but offer the shorter chain fatty acid (alpha linolenic acid) which the body can convert into the longer chain EPA or DHA used in the brain.

Insight

The conversion rate from the 'non-fish' fatty acids may be very low – less than one per cent for DHA and not much higher for EPA. Conversion is detrimentally affected by a diet high in saturated fats or too many omega 6 fatty acids, so if you are relying on fish-free sources of fatty acids, reduce your intake of saturated animal fats and vegetable oils/spreads rich in safflower or sunflower oil, as these foods are rich in omega 6 fats which will limit the conversion rate.

✓ *Use either linseed or rapeseed oil for salad dressings.*
✓ *Use olive oil for cooking.*

WHY ARE EPA AND DHA BETTER THAN A COD LIVER OIL SUPPLEMENT?

In the past we have commonly used cod liver oil for joint problems and for general health, but although cod liver oil is a fish oil, there are several reasons why EPA and DHA fish oils are a better supplement.

▶ *Cod liver oil capsules do not contain the same levels of EPA and DHA omega 3 oils, making them less effective than fish oil supplements which provide 1 g (1,000 mg) of EPA or DHA in a daily dose.*
▶ *Fish such as cod store much of their fat along with fat-soluble vitamins such as vitamin A in the liver; vitamin A is therefore present in most cod liver oil supplements. However, although vitamin A is essential in our diet, high intakes can be detrimental to our health so vitamin A supplementation is safer in the form of beta carotene. Good quality fish oil supplements may, however, contain vitamin E, another fat-soluble vitamin that will help to maintain the stability of the fatty acids in the fish oil supplement.*
▶ *Lastly, as the liver is an organ of detoxification, high levels of contaminants such as mercury or polychlorinated biphenyls (PCBs) may be present in cod liver oil supplements, although these pollutants can occur in any fish oil supplement even if the oils have been extracted from the flesh of the fish rather than the liver.*

HOW MUCH EPA OR DHA DO WE NEED?

The Scientific Advisory Committee on Nutrition Report (2006) advises that we should consume at least 450 mg of omega 3 fatty acids every day, with 500 mg/day being a figure that is generally accepted as a healthy intake. However, some people have been shown to respond well to intakes of 1,000 mg (1 g) or more daily, particularly those suffering with health conditions such as those listed below:

▶ *dementia*
▶ *attention deficit hyperactivity disorder*
▶ *depression*
▶ *anxiety*
▶ *autism*

- *dyslexia*
- *arthritis*
- *eczema*
- *heart disease.*

If you suffer with any of these health conditions and think you may benefit from more fatty acids, the first step is to adjust your diet so that you are consuming more essential fatty acids.

If you eat fish …

… consume between one to two portions of fish each week (or up to four portions if you are not pregnant or breastfeeding). One of these portions should be oily fish (or two if you are eating more fish).

Oily fish

Salmon	Pilchards
Mackerel	Tuna
Trout	Swordfish
Herring	Kipper
Sardines	Anchovies

White/non-oily fish

Cod	Whiting
Haddock	Halibut
Coley	Skate
Plaice	Rock salmon
Lemon sole	Dover sole

If you don't eat fish …

… it may be difficult to consume enough linolenic acid as large amounts of this essential fatty acid are only found in foods such as linseeds, linseed oil, walnuts and green leafy vegetables, and the conversion rate into the longer fatty acids isn't always high. A fish oil supplement could therefore help. Check how much EPA and DHA is included in each capsule – you may find that you need to take a few capsules to consume 500 mg daily, so look out for fish oil supplements that provide 500 mg in just one or two capsules.

If this sample omega 3-rich meal plan looks very different from your normal diet, it's worth changing the foods that you eat before you reach for the supplements ...

HAVE AN OMEGA 3-RICH DAY!

Breakfast	Omega 3 fortified egg on wholemeal toast and fresh orange juice
Snack	Nut/seed bar containing linseeds/flaxseeds
Lunch	Fresh (or tinned) sardines with a large green leafy salad, cherry tomatoes, beetroot and carrot with new potatoes
Snack	Yoghurt (dairy or soya) topped with mixed seeds (yoghurt with added omega 3 oils would boost intake)
Dinner	Salmon with broccoli, sweet potato and carrots; or spinach and sweet potato risotto drizzled with omega 3 oil

Nutrients for brain power

As we age our cognitive function is directly linked with our nutritional status. In short, a healthy diet sustains a healthy mind. Several vitamins and minerals have been repeatedly linked with mental and emotional function, linking deficiencies with the following conditions:

- *anti-social behaviour*
- *hyperactivity*
- *depressed mood*
- *anxiety*
- *insomnia*
- *irritability*
- *Alzheimer's disease*
- *dementia*
- *and a lower IQ.*

THE B VITAMINS

As well as aiding in nutrient metabolism, each of the B group of vitamins has essential roles, several of which are integrally linked with mental function.

Vitamin B_1 mimics and maximizes the action of an important neurotransmitter involved in memory function called acetylcholine. In several double-blind, placebo controlled studies, thiamine supplementation improved mood and feelings of well-being, with subjects also reporting increased clear-headedness and faster reaction times. Symptoms affecting the brain and mental function have been linked with a number of the B vitamins.

Symptoms of vitamin B_1 (thiamine) deficiency:

- *irritability*
- *inactivity*
- *fatigue*
- *decreased self-confidence*
- *introversion*
- *depression.*

Symptoms of vitamin B_3 (niacin) deficiency:

- *mental fatigue*
- *apathy*
- *memory loss*

- *psychosis*
- *dementia.*

Symptoms of vitamin B$_6$ (pyridoxine) deficiency:

- *pre-menstrual syndrome*
- *autism*
- *depression.*

Symptoms of vitamin B$_{12}$ (cyanocobalamine) deficiency:

- *impaired mental function*
- *depression (particularly in the elderly).*

Insight

Vitamin B$_{12}$ is stored in the liver and levels decline with age – deficiency is found in up to 42 per cent of people aged 65 and over. In one study, complete recovery was observed in over 60 per cent of cases where mental impairment was due to vitamin B$_{12}$ deficiency, highlighting the importance of a healthy, nutritious diet.

FOLIC ACID

A high percentage of depressed patients have been found to have poor folate (folic acid) status. Folic acid is involved in producing neurotransmitters, the chemical messengers in the brain, and without ample levels of neurotransmitters, our mental function quickly becomes impaired. A number of studies have reported an association between deficiencies of folate or vitamin B$_{12}$ and psychiatric conditions such as dementia and depression.

Relatively low levels of each of the B vitamins are required to maintain good health and these are found – usually together – in a wide range of foods. Make sure you base each meal around

these foods and it is unlikely you will have a deficiency of
B vitamins:

- ✓ *vegetables*
- ✓ *whole grains*
- ✓ *fruit*
- ✓ *beans*
- ✓ *pulses*
- ✓ *eggs*
- ✓ *meat*
- ✓ *fish*
- ✓ *dairy produce.*

ZINC

Zinc deficiency is widespread, and becomes increasingly common as
we age. It is required for many anti-oxidant enzymes, so a deficiency
may result in higher levels of cellular damage, including oxidative
damage to brain cells. Zinc levels in the brains of those suffering with
Alzheimer's disease are often found to be considerably lower, and it
has been suggested that zinc deficiency may be a significant causative
factor. Supplementation of this mineral in Alzheimer patients
has yielded unbelievable results in some patients, with significant
improvements in up to 80 per cent of patients in some studies.

Insight: Do you have a zinc deficiency?

Common symptoms of zinc deficiency include the following:

- ▶ *white specks on nails*
- ▶ *stretch marks*
- ▶ *poor blood sugar control*
- ▶ *mood swings and depression.*

SOUND FAMILIAR?

Several studies have linked psychological symptoms to low zinc
levels. In one study of 174 older adults, 71 per cent of subjects with
zinc deficiency displayed a higher value on a depression test against
29 per cent of subjects with a normal zinc value.

OTHER NUTRIENTS

Many nutrients are involved in healthy mental function, and several anti-oxidant vitamins and minerals are needed to help prevent oxidative damage that can lead to brain cell degeneration. Therefore, rather than supplement with any one nutrient, it is recommended that unless you are following a treatment plan prescribed by a qualified practitioner, a multi-vitamin, multi-mineral supplement is the best way to increase nutrient intake alongside a healthy diet. In most cases of mental impairment, best results following nutrient supplementation are observed when symptoms have been present for less than six months – when symptoms have been present for longer, it takes more time to correct nutrient deficiencies or imbalances and, in some cases, the deficiencies may never fully recover, particularly in dementia and Alzheimer's disease. Even better than correcting deficiencies swiftly is preventing them in the first place: prevention is always better than cure!

Try these nutrient-rich foods to keep your brain in tip top condition.

For zinc:

- ✓ *Add pumpkin seeds and wheat germ to cereals and yoghurts.*
- ✓ *Enjoy oysters when eating out.*
- ✓ *Eat dark cuts of meat (leg rather than breast) as they contain more zinc.*

For vitamin B_1:

- ✓ *Add a seed mix to fortified cereals.*
- ✓ *For a quick snack, eat beans on wholemeal toast.*
- ✓ *Enjoy mixed beans in chillies, curries and casseroles.*

For folic acid:

- ✓ *Eat raspberries with fortified breakfast cereals.*
- ✓ *Always add spinach, rocket or watercress to salad sandwiches.*
- ✓ *Enjoy salads with salmon or cottage cheese.*

For vitamin B$_6$:

✓ *Add a seed mix to fortified cereals.*
✓ *Enjoy trout poached with vegetables.*
✓ *Add grilled strips of meat to stir fries.*

For vitamin B$_{12}$:

✓ *Breakfast on eggs on toast.*
✓ *Add tofu to stir fries.*
✓ *Include yoghurts as a healthy snack.*

The effect of low blood sugar levels

Although specific nutrients such as omega 3 fatty acids, vitamin B$_1$ or zinc are specifically linked to mental function, there are more general areas of nutrition which have just as much effect upon our mood and performance. Blood sugar levels are a fundamental requirement for brain function – glucose is the brain's only fuel source (apart from ketones, which circulate during carbohydrate starvation) – which explains why we lose concentration and become irritated whenever blood sugar levels begin to drop.

Research with school children has shown improvements in attention, problem solving and memory when comparing the effect of breakfast versus no breakfast.

To maintain a constant source of glucose for the brain, always eat breakfast to elevate blood glucose levels first thing in the morning, and eat regular meals to maintain a constant energy source.

Insight: Five fast ways to get fuel to your brain cells!
1 *Use a sports energy drink.*
2 *Mix your own energy drink with equal amounts of juice and water.*
3 *Enjoy a few slices of juicy watermelon.*

(Contd)

4   *Get a quick fix with jam on white bread toasted.*
5   *There's always the good old caffeine fix – but try green tea instead of coffee.*

Missing any meal usually results in consuming caffeine or sugary snacks to elevate blood sugar, but whilst these may increase glucose levels for brain function, they offer no nutrients for optimal mental function, and the resulting blood sugar crash following an extreme high is detrimental to concentration, mental aptitude and performance.

Case study

Michelle had suffered with anxiety, mood swings and depression for several years, but she had never linked it to her diet. Whilst travelling to Thailand she stayed on a remote island. The diet was very plain, mostly rice and a few vegetables, but she soon realized that her mood swings had completely disappeared without her regular caffeine and sugar fix. A return to the UK and to her bad dietary habits confirmed her suspicions when her mood swings returned with the daily cappuccino and muffin!

Dietary benefits for specific mental health conditions

It's clear to see that many nutrients in our diet affect the way that we feel and think. Although a healthy balanced diet will generally help to reduce the risk of deficiency symptoms, and improve existing health conditions, there are some nutrients that are specifically linked with particular mental conditions.

INSOMNIA

There can be several diet-related causes of insomnia:

▶ *too much caffeine through the day*
▶ *alcohol affecting sleep patterns*
▶ *low blood sugar levels throughout the night which wakes you up*

- *lack of relaxing neurotransmitters (chemical messengers in the brain) that promote sleep*
- *mineral imbalances (e.g. too much copper and not enough zinc).*

Caffeine affects some people more than others, and consuming caffeine-rich substances through the day can significantly affect the onset or quality of sleep. Equally, although many people think that alcohol induces sleep, it actually disrupts sleep patterns and is best avoided if insomnia is present.

One cause of insomnia specifically linked to diet is an unbalanced ratio between the minerals zinc and copper. Too much copper and/or too little zinc in the diet over a prolonged period can cause heightened brain activity which keeps us awake. Certain lifestyle factors can increase our need for zinc – if any of these apply to you, or if you have stretch marks or white specks on your nails, you may need more zinc in your diet.

Common lifestyle factors that deplete zinc:

- *long-term use of the contraceptive pill*
- *smoking*
- *alcohol consumption*
- *chronic stress*
- *a vegetarian diet.*

Insight

Check whether you have copper water pipes in the home or are using copper pans to cook with, as these can both increase your intake of copper.

Without a rich source of zinc in the diet (oysters, whole grains, pumpkin seeds, meat and offal) zinc can become depleted. Foods rich in copper include offal, seafood and mushrooms, although a zinc deficiency is more likely to create a poor zinc:copper ratio than consuming too much copper in foods. Simply limiting your intake of copper-rich foods and ensuring that you consume plenty of zinc in your diet may be all you need to do to calm your mind down enough to get to sleep.

Another cause of insomnia can be low levels of iron, which may or may not be low enough to cause pallor, lack of energy or anaemia. As with zinc, iron is found in meats, although eating plenty of beans and pulses, grains and dark green leafy vegetables can provide enough iron for vegetarians or vegans. It is worth ensuring that you include rich sources of these minerals in a healthy balanced diet, but seek the advice of a health professional before rushing off to supplement these minerals, as taking any nutrients in isolation can create an imbalance of other nutrients.

Restless legs syndrome may cause insomnia. It is characterized by a compulsion to keep moving the legs, and has circulatory causes but may respond to additional iron, folic acid and vitamin E in the diet. A multi-vitamin, multi-mineral containing these nutrients in conjunction with a diet containing ample protein, whole grains and green leafy vegetables is a good place to begin if this is disrupting your sleep. If you suffer from insomnia, adjust your diet as follows and see if your sleep patterns improve.

Top ten tips for sleep

1 *Reduce or stop drinking coffee and tea, fizzy drinks and eating chocolate.*
2 *Avoid drinking alcohol.*
3 *Eat regularly throughout the day to keep blood sugar levels at a constant level.*
4 *Eat a supper rich in slow-release carbohydrates such as oats to keep blood sugar elevated through the night – a drop in glucose stimulates changes in hormone levels, which wake you.*
5 *Avoid quick-release carbohydrates during the day which may be causing nocturnal low blood sugar (hypoglycaemia).*
6 *Include protein foods in your evening meal and supper – these will slow down glucose absorption and also provide the amino acid tryptophan, which can be converted into serotonin to help you sleep.*

7 *Combine slow-release carbohydrates to promote serotonin production with foods rich in tryptophan in supper snacks to promote relaxation and sleep.*

8 *Make sure you have enough zinc in the diet to suppress high copper levels, as copper heightens brain activity and can keep you awake. Zinc-rich foods include meat, seafood, whole grains and pumpkin seeds.*

9 *Ensure that you include enough iron, folic acid and vitamin E in your diet to avoid restless legs syndrome. Find iron in meat or green leafy vegetables, folic acid in raspberries or salmon, and vitamin E in nuts and vegetable oils.*

10 *Other minerals known to enhance relaxation and sleep are calcium and magnesium; both minerals are found in milk, hence the remedy of a milky drink to encourage sleep.*

PRE-MENSTRUAL TENSION (PMT)

There are several dietary factors that have been linked to pre-menstrual tension or pre-menstrual syndrome. If you suffer with this condition, try the dietary adjustments discussed on the next page and see if you feel the benefit. Remember, dietary changes may take a few months to take effect.

Do you need a blood sugar fix?
Hypoglycaemia (low blood sugar) and cravings for sweet foods and refined carbohydrates are common at this time of the month, as changing hormone levels affect insulin production, which in turn affects blood sugar levels.

You can help to stabilize blood sugar levels by:

- *eating slow-release, low GI carbohydrates (oats and beans)*
- *avoiding or reducing stimulants (caffeine, alcohol and nicotine)*
- *reducing high GI, quick-release carbohydrates (sugary foods)*
- *eating at least three meals daily with snacks in between*
- *and filling up on wholesome foods that are rich in the nutrients which help to control blood sugar levels (magnesium, zinc, chromium, manganese and calcium) – beans and pulses, vegetables, rice, oats, nuts, seeds, fish and lean meats.*

Reaching for the chocolate? Maybe you need more serotonin?
Levels of 'feel good' hormones called endorphins drop prior to menstruation which can cause nausea, moodiness and increased agitation. In particular, serotonin levels decrease, affecting mood and increasing sensitivity to pain; women who experience PMS have been found to have lower levels of serotonin in their brains prior to menstruation.

Serotonin is formed from an essential amino acid called tryptophan. See pages 215 and 216 for a list of tryptohan-rich foods and carbohydrate combinations.

Maybe a fatty acid deficiency is to blame...
Pain and tenderness may also be increased by an imbalance in hormone-like substances called prostaglandins. These compounds are dependant upon the correct balance of essential fatty acids, so a deficiency of either omega 3 fatty acids or any of the nutrients which enable conversion of omega 6 fatty acids into

anti-inflammatory prostaglandins may result in inflammation or increased blood clotting.

If you suffer with abdominal cramps, breast tenderness, headaches, constipation or diarrhoea, you may benefit from the following dietary adjustments or from fatty acid supplementation, as this has improved the condition in some women.

Re-adjusting your fatty acid profile
- ✓ *Swap meat for fish.*
- ✓ *Snack on linseeds and walnuts instead of crisps and sweets.*
- ✓ *Use linseed oil or rapeseed oil for salad dressings, and rapeseed oil or olive oil for cooking instead of safflower or sunflower oils.*

Is it due to low vitamin or mineral levels?
Low levels of zinc, magnesium, vitamin B_6 and vitamin E have all been connected to this condition, and each of the aforementioned causes of pre-menstrual tension and/or pre-menstrual syndrome may be due to micronutrient deficiencies – in the end, it often comes back to having a healthy diet!

Follow any of the healthy eating plans in this book for a healthy, balanced diet that will contain ample levels of all of these nutrients. A multi-vitamin, multi-mineral supplement will help you to correct deficiencies quicker when taken in conjunction with a healthy diet, although mineral deficiencies in particular may take a number of months to correct.

Insight: Quick fix whilst making long-term corrections
Some symptoms of PMS such as low blood sugar levels may be improved quite quickly, but mineral deficiencies or a fatty acid imbalance can take a while to correct. Make the dietary adjustments that relate to your symptoms, but in the meantime, for a quick fix try the following:

1 *Eat slow-release carbohydrates with protein at each meal.*
2 *Invest in a multi-mineral, multi-vitamin.*
3 *Try supplementing with fatty acids.*

Basic nutrition to help pre-menstrual tension or pre-menstrual syndrome

▶ *Eat low GI carbohydrates (those that are absorbed slowly) to help control blood glucose levels and choose unrefined whole grains to increase your intake of essential nutrients.*

▶ *Eat small amounts of protein at each meal to help slow down the release of glucose into the bloodstream – this will help to stabilize blood glucose levels and the protein also provides many micronutrients.*

▶ *Swap meat for fish for a favourable fatty acid intake that will increase anti-inflammatory pathways and reduce swelling and pain. Alternatively, introduce linseeds, linseed oil and walnuts into your diet as these all provide linolenic acid which promotes anti-inflammatory reactions.*

....

Insight: Evening primrose oil or omega 3 fatty acids?

If dietary adjustments do not improve your PMT, consider supplementing with omega 3 fatty acids or evening primrose oil. These are different types of fatty acid with different roles, and you may need one or both of them. You could try just one of these supplements first to see if it improves your condition, although some supplements do contain them both and you can take them both together.

....

ATTENTION DEFICIT DISORDER, HYPERACTIVITY, DYSLEXIA, AUTISM ...

Although these are all separate conditions, their occurrence often overlaps in families and in individuals, the conditions share many of the symptoms and they often respond well to the same dietary adjustments. In particular, scientific evidence suggests that fatty acid deficiencies or imbalances may contribute to a wide range of behavioural and learning disorders.

Fatty acids

Essential fatty acids and long chain fatty acids are often lacking in our diet and a high intake of saturated, trans, hydrogenated, and even omega 6 fatty acids compounds the effects of this deficiency. There are several studies as well as a host of epidemiological findings that show positive results in hyperactivity, anti-social behaviour and cognitive function following fatty acid supplementation. In the largest trial to date supplementing children with ADHD (attention deficit hyperactivity disorder) with polyunsaturated fatty acids, positive results were published in the Journal of Developmental & Behavioural Paediatrics (2007), showing significant improvements in core ADHD symptoms such as inattention, restlessness, hyperactivity and impulsivity in almost half of the 132 children in the trial compared to the placebo group.

A 14-year study examining links between childhood diet and teenage anti-social behaviour illustrated a 51 per cent rise in aggression at age 17 in those who ate a poor diet with low levels of zinc, iron, B vitamins and protein. These deficiencies were linked to poor brain development, which led to a low IQ, resulting in anti-social behaviour. In another study, IQ was found to be 25 points lower in children who ate a diet rich in refined carbohydrates.

Whole foods versus junk foods
A processed food diet will be low in the nutrients that we need to feed our brain; symptoms of deficiency include irritability, aggression, inability to concentrate and depression. In addition to being devoid of micronutrients (minerals and vitamins), added sugar also creates fluctuations in blood glucose levels, contributing to hyperactivity, mood swings and poor concentration.

Numerous studies and reviews of controlled trials have shown that the behaviour of hyperactive children improves when artificial food colourings are eliminated from their diet. The average improvement is around one third to one half of the improvement typically associated with medication for attention deficit hyperactivity disorder.

Additives
A report published by *The Food Magazine* in 2007 revealed that several colourings and preservatives regularly used in food

and drinks have to carry health warnings if they are added to medicines. Warnings include allergic and hyperactivity reactions for the following additives, which are commonly used in products such as cakes, sweets and soft drinks:

- *tartrazine*
- *sunset yellow* } *(these are artificial colourings)*
- *ponceau red*
- *sodium benzoate*
- *sodium dioxide* } *(these are preservatives)*
- *sodium metabisulphite*

A Southampton University study found that a quarter of three year olds illustrated hyperactivity and tantrums after consuming certain colourings and preservatives commonly added to foods; behaviour that many parents recognize in their children. Many additives are outlawed in other countries including the USA and Japan, but are still added to cheap, processed foods available in the UK.

Insight: Not all additives are bad...

Some E numbers are natural compounds, such as anti-oxidants including vitamin C (ascorbic acid) or curcumin derived from the yellow spice turmeric, providing colouring to foods. Check out a full list of E numbers on www.ukfoodguide.net/enumeric to see what you need to avoid.

Good nutrition for young brains!

- *Try to avoid foods with artificial additives and a long list of E numbers as much as possible (see Chapter 9 for tips on how to change your children's diet).*
- *Stabilize blood sugar to help avoid hyperactivity by introducing slow-release carbohydrates such as porridge and beans into the diet. This will reduce lack of concentration when blood sugar levels drop again.*
- *Including protein foods such as eggs, fish or meat in each meal also slows down glucose release into the bloodstream and will provide a range of nutrients for health.*

- *Include fish or vegetable sources of alpha-linolenic acid (linseeds, walnuts) in the diet to provide a source of long chain polyunsaturated fatty acids for the brain.*

SAMPLE MENUS FOR A YOUNG EINSTEIN!

Breakfast

- *Milky porridge with added mixed seeds, chopped walnuts and fruit*
- *Omega 3 fortified boiled egg with toasted wholemeal bread soldiers*
- *Scrambled/poached egg (fortified) on wholemeal toast with baked beans*

Lunch

- *Tuna or salmon salad sandwich with wholemeal bread*
- *Corn tortilla wrap with turkey, spinach, bean sprouts and avocado*
- *Sardines on wholemeal toast*

Supper

- *Turkey or salmon risotto*
- *Vegetable chilli with brown rice*
- *Home made fish cakes/good quality fish fingers with peas and roasted potato skins.*

DEMENTIA

In the same way that free radicals create cell damage in other parts of the body causing ageing, the same oxidative damage occurs in the neurons (nerve cells) in the brain (Check out Chapter 6 for more information on oxidative damage and ageing). Dementia is usually a result of several degenerative changes in the brain over a period of time.

Our brains contain large amounts of fatty tissue, partly to insulate the nerve cells that carry electrical impulses from one cell to another. The reason why 'fish makes you brainy' (an old wives' tale) is that it is the long chain polyunsaturated fats found in fish which form much of the structure and function of the brain. However, being polyunsaturated means that these fatty acids are at greater risk of oxidative damage.

Meals rich in anti-oxidants and long chain fatty acids

Breakfast	Kedgeree – smoked mackerel with brown rice and wilted spinach with a glass of orange juice
Lunch	Peppered mackerel with a green leafy salad and grated carrot
Dinner	Tuna steak with olive oil roasted squash, sweet potato and carrots, served with broccoli

Prevention of oxidative damage is better than cure, so follow these simple dietary tips to maintain good mental health and prevent oxidative damage ...

1 *Eat fish regularly.*
2 *Include anti-oxidants to protect the long chain fatty acids.*

Anti-oxidants such as vitamin E and zinc have created beneficial results with dementia and Alzheimer's disease.

ALZHEIMER'S DISEASE

Alzheimer's is thought to be caused by the build up of amyloid plaques in conjunction with increased oxidative damage, causing brain cell degeneration and mental ageing. There is also thought to be a genetic factor involved, but a number of nutritional elements have been shown to have a significant effect upon the occurrence and severity of Alzheimer's disease.

Fish

Docosahexaenoic acid (DHA) has been shown to be deficient in the brains of Alzheimer's patients when compared with individuals of the same age without this degenerative disease. In addition, preliminary studies have shown low serum DHA to be a significant risk factor for the development of Alzheimer's, also commonly found in ageing individuals with reduced cognitive function. DHA is one of the long chain fatty acids found in fish, so it makes sense to include several portions of fish in our diet, especially as we age.

Fruit and vegetables

Foods rich in anti-oxidants may help to prevent oxidative damage occurring, hence preventing the onset of conditions such as Alzheimer's. Some foods are not only rich in anti-oxidant nutrients, such as vitamin C, but also contain phytonutrients which have powerful anti-oxidant properties (see Chapter 3 for more information on phytonutrients).

Insight

Drink unsweetened red grape juice or cranberry juice every day.

In one study of 1836 adults, there was no apparent association found with the onset of Alzheimer's and dietary intake of vitamins E, C, or beta-carotene, but there was a reduced incidence in those who drank juices at least three times per week compared with those who drank juices less often than once per week. This was thought to be due to the polyphenol (phytonutrient) content of fruit and vegetable juices.

The aluminium theory

Although there is no conclusive proof that aluminium causes Alzheimer's disease, it has been proven that as we age blood aluminium levels increase, and those suffering with Alzheimer's disease have significantly higher levels of aluminium in their brains than normal. The most effective way to avoid this is to limit our intake of aluminium as follows:

- ✗ *Don't use aluminium pots and pans.*
- ✗ *Avoid using aluminium foil to wrap food.*
- ✗ *Choose anti-perspirants that don't contain aluminium.*
- ✗ *Avoid the use of antacids for heartburn.*
- ✗ *Although this mineral occurs naturally in water, some water companies add it as a water treatment, so it may be worth checking with your local supplier, or swapping to bottled water.*
- ✗ *Don't add salt to food as aluminium is sometimes added to table salt.*

Nutrition to help prevent dementia and Alzheimer's disease

- ▶ *Swap meat for fish and include different types of fish in your diet two to four times weekly.*
- ▶ *Include foods rich in plant-based omega 3 fatty acids in your diet, such as linseeds, linseed oil and walnuts. This is especially important if you don't eat fish.*
- ▶ *Make sure you eat at least five servings of fresh fruit and vegetables daily to maximize your anti-oxidant intake to help prevent oxidative damage to brain cells.*
- ▶ *Consume fruits and vegetables rich in polyphenols, anthocyanidins and anti-oxidants, in particular berries, red grapes and cherries.*
- ▶ *Drink green tea to increase anti-oxidant intake.*

Insight: Remember the anti-oxidants?

Colour your meals with these anti-oxidant rich foods …

Get vitamin C from green leafy vegetables, peppers, citrus fruit and kiwi, vitamin E by including avocado, olive oil, nuts and seeds in your diet, and beta carotene from orange-coloured fruits and vegetables.

DEPRESSION

Clinically depressed people often have lower levels of omega 3 fatty acids in their blood and several studies have shown that supplementing a diet with omega 3 fatty acids can relieve depression. Eating more omega 3 fatty acids leads to a higher volume of grey matter in the areas of the brain associated with emotional arousal and regulation; these fats also enhance mood.

Blood sugar blues

Something as simple as low blood sugar affects our mood, even to the extent of depression. Reducing your intake of stimulants and sugary foods may have a significant effect upon your mood and it is such a simple (though not always easy!) thing to do. Although foods and drinks that provide a quick surge of energy (which includes the flood of glucose that goes to your brain) and a lift in mood seem to do a good job, this 'high' in blood sugar may be followed by a 'low' as insulin is released to reduce the high level of glucose in the bloodstream.

These fluctuations in blood sugar can become more pronounced over a period of time, creating blood sugar conditions that can affect your mood. You can often feel when your blood sugar levels are low due to symptoms such as:

▶ *feeling hungry*
▶ *craving sugary foods or caffeine*
▶ *feeling moody or fed up*
▶ *feeling anxious or irritable*
▶ *inability to concentrate*
▶ *your head may feel 'fuzzy'*
▶ *feeling faint or dizzy*
▶ *spots before the eyes or inability to focus*
▶ *shaking*
▶ *you may even faint if your blood sugar drops too low.*

Insight: Keep a food and mood diary

Jot down everything that you eat and drink for a week and also note how you're feeling. See if you can spot any of the symptoms of low blood sugar listed above – if you do, this may be causing mood swings or even depression, as well as creating problems with blood sugar regulation.

Blood sugar conditions

Highs and lows in our blood sugar levels are normal to an extent, but if we continue causing extreme fluctuations in blood sugar, we can create chronic conditions that often occur prior to diabetes.

FASTING HYPOGLYCAEMIA (LOW BLOOD SUGAR)

This means you have a low blood glucose level for most of the time, which will lead to poor concentration, mind 'fuzziness' and depressed mood.

REACTIVE HYPOGLYCAEMIA

Elevated blood sugar levels with hyperactivity or irritability followed by a severe low with depressed mood are indicative of this condition, which can also make you feel faint and dizzy when blood sugar levels drop.

If this sounds familiar and you think your blood sugar levels may be linked to your moods, try keeping a food and mood diary – it will help you to see which foods affect you the most and allow you to monitor your progress. A simple symbol to indicate how you're feeling each morning, lunchtime and evening will help you to measure how you're doing – simply add up the number of 'smiley faces' at the end of each week to see if your diet is improving your mood!

Feeling great ☺   Feeling okay ☺   Bad day! ☹

Supplements to help mental function

Naturally, there are a range of nutrients that may enhance mental health, but an individual's requirements will depend on current and past dietary habits, lifestyle and genetics. It cannot be presumed that any supplement will help alleviate a symptom until the health condition is diagnosed and/or a full nutritional and health assessment has taken place. The first steps towards better health should always be dietary adjustments, which may remove the need for any dietary supplementation. However, a good multi-vitamin, multi-mineral preparation including, or in addition to, anti-oxidants can be a useful support for a healthy diet and will encourage better general health in addition to supporting mental function. There are, however, some supplements that are often linked with mental and emotional improvements.

GINGKO BILOBA

Gingko biloba has been used as a medicinal herb for thousands of years. A well-known herb, it is often used to improve memory and to help reduce the symptoms of dementia. It works by dilating (widening) the cerebral arteries and improving blood circulation to the brain. Gingko biloba contains several different active compounds, including flavonoids, which are anti-oxidants, helping to counteract free radical damage in all tissues, including those of the brain and cerebral circulation.

Gingko biloba has been known to enhance functions such as:

▶ *memory*
▶ *learning*
▶ *intellect*
▶ *emotion.*

ST JOHN'S WORT

Another herb used to improve mental function is St. John's Wort, which has several medicinal uses, but is commonly taken to reduce insomnia and depression. It is thought to work through increasing the concentration or effectiveness of serotonin in the brain, enhancing a feeling of well-being.

PHOSPHATIDYL SERINE

This nutrient determines the fluidity and function of cell membranes in the brain. The richest source in the diet is soya, but food does not provide enough of this nutrient, and a healthy body usually manufactures what it needs. However, if we lack essential fatty acids, folic acid or vitamin B_{12} in the diet, our ability to manufacture phosphatidyl serine is affected. With advancing age we seem to become less able to form this nutrient, and low levels are specifically associated with impaired mental function and dementia.

Insight

In some studies, tests with phosphatidyl serine supplementation have reportedly 'turned the (mental) clock back 12 years', giving renewed cognitive function similar to that of a 52 year old to someone aged 64!

Although supplementation with this nutrient may be useful, the first steps are to ensure a diet rich in the nutrients we need to naturally manufacture phosphatidyl serine in the body – fill up on these foods and see if it makes a difference to your memory:

- ▶ *Eat fish, nuts, seeds (especially linseeds), and nut and seed oils (especially linseed oil) for the essential fatty acids you've already read so much about.*
- ▶ *Folic acid is found in foods such as raspberries, green leafy vegetables, beans, salmon, cottage cheese and fortified breakfast cereals.*
- ▶ *Vitamin B_{12} can be found in eggs, meat, fish, dairy, tofu and fortified cereals.*

EPA/DHA (OMEGA 3 FATTY ACIDS)

If fish isn't your idea of a tasty meal or snack, you may benefit from supplementing with fish oils. Look for a supplement that provides 500 mg to 1,000 mg (1 g) of EPA or a mixture of EPA and DHA in one or two capsules. Some individuals may benefit from taking a combination of fish oil with evening primrose oil – this will depend upon your particular symptoms, so consulting with a nutritional therapist will help to identify your individual fatty acid requirements. Some reputable supplement companies are included in the 'Taking it further' section at the end of this book.

THINGS TO REMEMBER

Although these things are all great changes to make to your diet, if you try to change everything at once, you may feel worse before you feel better! This is particularly true if you are addicted to stimulants such as caffeine, nicotine or alcohol, so you might try reducing all of these gradually, or cutting them out one at time.

- *Avoid or limit stimulants such as alcohol, nicotine and caffeine.*

- *Avoid sugars and refined carbohydrate foods such as biscuits, cakes and white bread for a few days and see how your mood is affected.*

- *Fill the gaps left by adding slow-release, wholesome beans, pulses, vegetables and brown rice.*

- *Eat regularly throughout the day.*

- *Include protein foods at each meal to help slow down blood glucose absorption and provide essential nutrients.*

- *Fill up on nutrient-rich foods to feed your brain – lean meats and fish, whole grains such as brown rice and oats, beans and pulses, and lots of fruits and vegetables. A balanced diet will help to create a balanced mood.*

- *Choose specific foods for enhanced mental function – for example, fish will provide omega 3 fatty acids and meat, offal, oysters, whole grains and pumpkin seeds are rich sources of zinc.*

- *Include tryptophan-rich foods in your diet (turkey, chicken, avocado, banana, broccoli and spinach) to maximize formation of the feel good hormone serotonin!*

- *Food allergies can be linked with poor mood and depression, so try excluding common allergens such as wheat, dairy produce and eggs from your diet for a few days and see how you feel. An improvement in mood may indicate that you've found the cause of your symptoms.*

- *If your diet is already good, supplementing with omega 3 fatty acids may help. You are advised to seek the help of a qualified practitioner for the best supplement prescription to suit you.*

9

Healthy eating for the family

In this chapter you will learn:
- *simple ways to boost the nutrient content of meals*
- *healthy recipes for breakfast, lunch and dinner*
- *how to cut corners to a healthy diet*
- *all about going organic.*

Eating healthily is much easier when the whole household is involved, with the added bonus of health benefits for the rest of the family, although they may not initially be as keen as you to give their eating habits an overhaul! But with increasing amounts of research linking health conditions to a poor diet and nutrient deficiencies, can you afford not to change the family palate? Simple changes such as introducing more fish and vegetables into the family diet can have a number of beneficial effects: from improving IQ and reducing behavioural difficulties in junior members of the family, to decreasing cholesterol levels and blood pressure in older family members.

Quick fixes for now ...

- ▶ *Swap meat for fish in at least one meal a week.*
- ▶ *Buy different types of fruit and make up a fruit salad.*
- ▶ *Swap white bread to wholemeal and white rice to brown.*

Small steps

Lifestyle changes are tough, and it can take up to 12 weeks for a new routine to become habitual. To get the rest of the family on board (or just to improve their health without them realizing!), make small changes to meals and eating habits to win the battle.

Sometimes all the persuasion (children) and selling of health benefits (husband or wife) seem to make no difference at all and, if this is the case, it may be time for some underhand cookery. This may be the only way to increase the nutrient content of your family's diet.

Insight: Hidden nutrients!

▶ *Add salad vegetables to sandwiches – don't put them on the side of the plate – they're likely to stay there!*

▶ *Make home-made coleslaw – not only will it taste better but it'll contain much more cabbage, carrot and onion than usual with less mayonnaise and additives – much healthier.*

▶ *Make home-made vegetable or fruit chutneys – another way to boost fruit and vegetable intake whilst reducing your family's consumption of salt, sugar and additives.*

▶ *Add frozen or chopped vegetables to sauces, curries, chilli, pasta and rice dishes ... it boosts the nutrient value, makes the meal look more colourful and taste more interesting, and takes no extra time if frozen vegetables are used.*

With a large proportion of family meals eaten at home or prepared at home, you have the maximum opportunity to have a positive impact on the family's nutrition and health. Think of how many breakfasts, lunches and dinners are eaten at home each week and you'll soon realize how much family meals contribute to the overall health of your family. If we typically eat breakfast, lunch and dinner each day – a total of 21 meals – which are the easiest meals for you to have a positive impact upon? Even if you can make breakfast a really healthy start to the day, that's one third (excluding snacks) of the meals your family will eat through the week … maybe you can send everyone off (including yourself) with a healthy lunch, or perhaps you want to concentrate on healthy dinners. Whatever the option, there are plenty of healthy eating ideas and tips to improve family nutrition … read on and choose what will suit you the best.

Healthy meal ideas

HAVE A HEALTHY START TO THE DAY

Fruit salad bowl

Eating fruit conjures up pictures of an apple, an orange or a banana for most of us, which isn't too inspiring! A bowl of different and exotic fruits placed in the middle of the table with different things to add can begin to seem like a trip to the 'help yourself ice cream factory' (well, not quite, but it's certainly more interesting than simply eating a piece of fruit). You can place different fruits in separate bowls to suit fussy eaters (group them together according to family likes and dislikes to save on the washing up) and putting together their own breakfast will increase the fun and ownership of a new breakfast.

INGREDIENTS FOR A FRUIT SALAD
Red grapes
Kiwi
A selection of berries – strawberries, blackberries, raspberries, blueberries
Blackcurrants or redcurrants
Chopped banana
Chopped apple or pear
Chopped mango, papaya or apricots
Greek yoghurt
Mixed seeds – sunflower seeds, linseeds and pumpkin seeds
Flaked almonds, chopped or whole hazelnuts or mixed nuts

Granola

Granola is a tasty and healthy alternative to normal breakfast cereals. Although you can buy it ready made, which would save you time, it won't be as healthy and is likely to be much more expensive. If you make a batch of granola you can keep it for a few days and also make cookies with it by sprinkling the granola mix over melted chocolate on a baking sheet (see recipes later on page 263). It's a healthy option because it is based upon oats and contains added nuts and seeds, and it tastes great because the oats are lightly toasted. It might be a nice weekend breakfast treat. Play around with the ingredient proportions until you find a mix and amount that suits you.

INGREDIENTS FOR GRANOLA

400 g oats
100 g barley or millet flakes (optional)
2 tbs sunflower seeds
2 tbs pumpkin seeds
2 tbs sesame seeds
2 tbs linseeds
200 g mixed chopped nuts or flaked almonds
50 g desiccated coconut (optional)
Honey

Preheat the oven to 175°C/Gas mark 4. Place all the ingredients in a bowl and mix thoroughly, coating the nuts, seeds and grains with honey. Spread the mixture out on a baking tray or baking sheet and lightly toast, mixing after 5–10 minutes to ensure even toasting. You can add un-toasted oats, seeds or nuts afterwards to bulk out the mixture and adjust the taste. Cool the mixture, then break up and put in an airtight container, ready to eat. As with the fruit salad, you could have different things on the table to add to the granola – try dried apricots or raisins, fresh fruit or yoghurt.

Porridge

Porridge provides a great start to the day as it has a low Glycaemic Index and is absorbed slowly, giving a sustained energy release throughout the morning and preventing snacking on sweet or sugary foods (see Chapter 7 to find out more about the Glycaemic Index). Oats have a number of benefits:

▶ *Including oats in the diet can help to lower cholesterol.*
▶ *Oats also provide a range of minerals and vitamins essential to good health.*
▶ *Oats have a low Glycaemic Index, releasing energy very slowly into the body.*

Unfortunately, porridge is often greeted with a grimace – from adults and children! Many of us will remember porridge as a 'gloopy' semolina-type mixture from our childhood days, but do try it again, as you might find you actually like it!

As well as its nutritious merits, porridge is a great family breakfast as it's quite versatile. You can microwave a sachet or serving of oats mixed with water or milk in a matter of minutes (great on school days), or make a pan of steaming porridge and serve it with a range of optional extras – have honey, yoghurt, cold milk, chopped banana, berries, mixed seeds and flaked almonds on the table for a really tasty breakfast.

Insight

Stewed fruit is a great option to add to porridge as it provides sweetness so you don't have to add sugar or honey to it to add taste (or salt!). You could stew the fruit whilst the porridge is cooking or do it the evening before – apples or rhubarb work well. Both apples and oats have been shown to reduce cholesterol levels, so if there is family history of elevated cholesterol, this is a great breakfast to eat regularly.

HEALTHY TUCK BOX IDEAS

Add pieces of fruit and vegetables to tuck boxes – celery, radish, tomatoes, chunks of fresh pepper and avocado, or slices of apple or pear ... it makes a sandwich meal look and taste much better and makes a change from the usual salad vegetables added to a sandwich. If this isn't enough to win against the tuck shop/chip shop/pie van, try some alternatives to the usual sandwich!

Pitta bread

Instead of a sandwich, fill pitta bread with shredded lettuce, onion, carrot and beetroot. You could spread some tasty hummus inside the pitta before adding your chosen ingredients, or add strips of cooked turkey or chicken, grated cheese or tinned tuna.

Tortilla wrap

If you're looking for a wheat-free alternative to the sandwich, tortilla wraps are just the job. Tortillas are made primarily from corn, but always check the packaging for any added wheat if you suffer from an allergy. Simply pile your ingredients in the middle and wrap the tortilla around the filling. You could use a rice salad, a Mediterranean mix with mozzarella cheese/tomato/avocado/rocket/pine nuts, or maybe a Waldorf salad – chopped apple, raisins and celery with any other salad vegetables you choose.

NO TIME TO MAKE LUNCH? NO PROBLEM, JUST MAKE EXTRA DINNER!

If you're short on time or motivation to create lunch at supper or breakfast time, make it easy on yourself by cooking an extra portion of dinner and creating tomorrow's lunch at the same time. Try these tasty, nutritious options to boost health and save time.

BROWN RICE RISOTTO (DINNER) AND RICE SALAD (LUNCH) FOR TWO

300 g organic brown rice
2 onions
2 cloves garlic
2 cups mushrooms
1 cup mixed peppers (frozen or fresh)
1 cup sweetcorn (frozen)
1 cup peas (frozen)
1 cup broccoli florets (fresh or frozen – if fresh you may wish to boil it briefly first)
1 tbs mixed seeds or pine nuts
Olive oil

Steam or boil 300 g of brown rice, or enough for four healthy servings as indicated on the packet. Meanwhile, chop the garlic, onion and mushroom and stir fry them in a little olive oil. Once browned, add the seeds and vegetables and cook through. Time the rice and stir-fried vegetables to be cooked at the same time, spoon the rice into the stir fry, mix thoroughly and serve. For a vegetarian dish providing complete protein just add any type of bean with the vegetables (use tinned baked beans for a quick and easy option, if using dried beans make sure you have pre-soaked and cooked them as required). Alternatively you can add chicken, turkey, salmon or tuna to the mix.

Don't forget to save one or two portions of your risotto for tomorrow's cold rice salad lunch. Easy!

BAKED POTATO (DINNER) AND POTATO SALAD (LUNCH) FOR TWO
4 medium potatoes plus an extra one for each lunch required
For potato salad (2 portions):
1 red onion
2 large tomatoes
A quarter of a cucumber
Half an avocado
2 beetroots
2 sticks of celery
2 tbs home-made coleslaw

This is a versatile option as you can cook a meal with baked potatoes or a supper snack of baked potatoes and simply bake an extra one for each lunch needed the following day. For potato salad, simple chop the cold potato up into bite size chunks and add tomato, cucumber, avocado, beetroot, red onion, celery and maybe some home-made coleslaw.

BEAN CASSEROLE (DINNER) AND MIXED BEAN SALAD (LUNCH) FOR TWO
Selection of beans/lentils, pre-soaked if necessary
2 large onions, chopped
2 cloves garlic, chopped
1–2 chillies, chopped (optional)

2 tsps turmeric
300 g organic brown rice
2 cups of fresh tomatoes
Vegetable stock cube
Selection of carrots, parsnips, broccoli, peas (2 cups in total)
Olive oil

Soak a selection of beans overnight before cooking them, or use tinned beans as an easier option. Whilst boiling the beans, brown the garlic and onion with a little oil in a casserole dish or large saucepan, then add the turmeric and/or chilli. Add the beans to the onion mix with approximately one litre of made up vegetable stock. Simmer for one hour or as required. Fresh or tinned tomatoes may be added if desired, along with two cupfuls of any other vegetables, lentils and other pulses not requiring pre-soaking. Serve with brown rice once the sauce has thickened and the beans have been boiled as directed on the packaging.

Put aside a portion of bean casserole to re-heat for lunch the next day, or mix with a tin of chickpeas for a cold bean salad – add a tortilla wrap for that Mexican feel!

VEGETABLE STEW – ENOUGH FOR STEW (DINNER) AND SOUP (LUNCH)
4 medium potatoes
4 carrots
4 parsnips
1 swede
2 onions
2 leeks
2 turnips
2 cups peas
(Meat or beans can be added as an optional extra)

Chop all the vegetables, add to a pan and simmer for 30–40 minutes, adding the peas towards the end if frozen. Add salt-free organic vegetable stock towards the end if desired, crushing the potatoes in the pan to thicken the gravy. Any type of bean/pulse may also be added to create a bean stew. Serve.

Any leftover stew can be re-heated the next day for another serving with a chunk of crusty bread, or put in a blender to create home-made vegetable soup which can be heated in the morning and taken to work or school in a flask.

NUTRITIOUS MEALS READY IN LESS THAN 20 MINUTES

Dinner is often the only time when a family has the opportunity to eat together, but it is also a time when you may be tired, late in from work, busy with taxi-driving duties for the kids, or simply not motivated to spend hours preparing a meal. Try out these quick, nutritious meals, taking no longer than 20 minutes to make – less if you use some of the 'cutting corners' tips below!

STIR FRY
Chop garlic, onion and mushrooms and stir fry them in a little olive oil. Once browned, add frozen vegetables and/or shredded spring cabbage and cook through. You can add a portion of grilled/baked fish or strips of chicken or turkey to the stir fry – the whole thing will take approximately 15 minutes.

MEDITERRANEAN-STYLE SALAD
Boil some new potatoes (optional for a more substantial meal), boil one egg per person, and parboil some asparagus spears (you could do this all in one pan). Meanwhile, throw a bag of spinach leaves into a large bowl and add a chopped avocado, chopped vine tomatoes and a handful of pine nuts with a drizzle of olive oil and some balsamic vinegar. Add the asparagus, eggs and potatoes once done (the eggs should be hard boiled), mix and serve. You can remove the asparagus and eggs from the pan first and add them to your salad if the potatoes need extra cooking.

Insight
Boil the kettle whilst the cooker ring and a small amount of water in a pan are heating up, then add boiling water to the preheated ring as required. This saves time and also preserves some of the vitamin C in the potatoes!

SALMON PARCELS

Place the required number of salmon fillets in a baking dish with a teaspoon of honey and a dessertspoon of soya sauce drizzled over each fillet (if you have the time, you could marinate the salmon in this mixture). You can either bake (approx. 20 minutes) or microwave (much quicker) the salmon. If baking, wrap the fillets in some foil so they cook in the foil parcel. Meanwhile, stir fry a red onion (cut in half and sliced rather than chopped for speed), some garlic, large mushrooms and already prepared mange tout, baby carrots and baby sweet corn. Add a little of the honey and soya sauce to the vegetables just before taking them out of the pan and serving with your 'marinated salmon'.

Cutting a few corners!

Okay, so optimum nutrition may sound like a great idea, but how realistic is it for the average person? We may like the idea of eating fresh, organic vegetables, or including beans and pulses in our diet because we've read so many times how good they are for us, but is it really do-able? The thing is, when we change our diet, we don't have to take a massive step from consuming mostly convenience foods to optimum nutrition – it's okay to take small steps and make small changes. In fact, we're more likely to stick with these smaller changes as they have less impact on our normal daily routines; a small step in the right direction is better than trying to be the perfect wife/mother/cook then reverting back to ready meals after three days!

SOUP TIP

We all know that packaged foods are less nutritious than fresh foods, but meeting optimum nutrition half way is better than changing nothing at all. Home-made soup made from fresh ingredients with no added salt is always going to be the healthiest soup option, but cartons of fresh soup are usually more nutritious than packet or tinned soups and will often provide one serving of vegetables.

Choose vegetable soups such as tomato, lentil, mixed vegetable or asparagus in a carton, opt for the one with the lowest salt content and avoid those with added cream.

SALAD TIP

Freshly prepared salad vegetables will be more nutritious, but if you haven't got time to prepare a salad there are lots of already prepared options available.

Choose from pre-washed and packaged salad leaves and packs of ready to eat salads, buy ready-grated carrot and beetroot, or opt for a Caesar salad and just add fresh ingredients to it ... avocado, cherry tomatoes, beetroot, etc. This way you increase your fresh vegetable intake but it's quick and easy to do.

FISH TIP

Fresh, oily fish will give you the omega 3 fatty acids you're after, but although white and tinned fish come in a poor second, they still provide a good source of protein, minerals and vitamins with some omega 3 fatty acids. Try these tips to increase your intake of fish and omega 3 fats.

Swap meat for peppered mackerel, tinned tuna or salmon on sandwiches, lunch on tinned sardines on toast instead of cheese, and buy frozen or pre-poached portions of salmon rather than having to prepare fresh fish.

VEGETABLE TIP

Washing, peeling and chopping vegetables is one of the most time consuming parts of preparing a meal. Although fresh is best, including plenty of vegetables in your diet is better than consuming none at all, so take it easy by buying already prepared options.

You can buy shredded cabbage or broccoli, cauliflower and carrots ready to steam or microwave in the bag, or just stock the freezer with frozen peas, sweetcorn, peppers and mixed vegetables for use as and when you need them. You can also buy already prepared vegetables ready to be stir-fried – it couldn't be simpler or quicker!

Get the family involved

You could say there are two foundations to successful, long-term healthy eating ... one is wanting to do it and the other is making it easy enough to do. Selling the benefits of eating certain foods to your family and presenting them with tasty meals that they enjoy eating will both increase the likelihood of the whole family enjoying a healthier diet. Another thing that can help win over children is increasing the ownership of a change in lifestyle or diet by getting them interested in healthy eating or involved in what they eat. They may be more likely to eat something if they have helped to grow or make it. There are a number of ways to do this:

1   *Get them involved in growing their own ... have your own vegetable plot, plant fruit trees, grow your own alfalfa sprouts or create a herb garden.*
2   *Make cooking and eating food a colourful, fun and enjoyable pastime rather than something that is simply 'something to eat'; have a colourful range of fruit available to add to breakfast cereals, buy different fruits for the fruit bowl, add colourful, different foods to tuck boxes or have them available in the fridge as snacks; get the children involved in cooking healthy muffins and flapjacks.*
3   *Link certain foods with health benefits that the family may relate to ... fish to increase your IQ, linseeds and walnuts to help improve inflammatory conditions such as eczema and asthma, or zinc-rich whole grains and pumpkin seeds to help with acne.*

Getting children involved in cooking has a number of benefits.

▶ *It gives them an interest and understanding of food and can help them to be less fussy about what they eat.*
▶ *It creates an opportunity to spend valuable family time together, making you feel less guilty about being in the kitchen whilst they're sitting watching TV!*
▶ *It helps to develop skills and nurture habits that will benefit your children's future eating habits.*

HEALTHY RECIPES FOR YOUNG COOKS!

VEGETABLE PIZZA FOR 4 PEOPLE
Use ready-made pizza bases to save time or make your own:

250 g durum wheat flour*
7 g sachet dried yeast
2 tbs olive oil
125 ml tepid/warm water
Variety of vegetable toppings ... onions, red onions, mushrooms,
  red, yellow and orange peppers, sweetcorn, spinach leaves,
  tomatoes
Tomato purée
Grated cheese or mozzarella

*225 g polenta can replace flour for a wheat-free option – cook the
polenta as per packet instructions, spread onto a baking tray and
place in a hot oven for 10 minutes to crisp the polenta base.

Deluxe version!
Mix the flour and yeast in a bowl and make a well in the centre.
Add the olive oil and water and work in the flour mix to make
dough. Transfer the dough onto a floured surface and knead
for approximately 10 minutes until it is smooth and stretchy.
Rub a little oil over the surface of the dough, put back in the
bowl, cover and leave in a warm place for about an hour for the
dough to 'rise'. Meanwhile, roast some vegetables in a little olive
oil for approximately 30 minutes (180°C/350°F/Gas mark 4) –
choose red onions, courgettes, peppers, aubergine and tomatoes
for a healthy Mediterranean flavour. Knead the risen dough and
roll it out on a floured surface to make the required number of
pizza bases. Preheat the oven to 220°C/425°F/Gas mark 7 whilst
you (and your helpers!) add your vegetable topping to the
pizzas.

Quick version!
Spread the lycopene-rich tomato purée over ready-made pizza
bases (see Chapter 3 for information on lycopene). Ask the

children to choose their vegetable toppings and place them on the pizza – the more vegetables the better for a healthy, tasty meal. Fresh or frozen peppers, peas, sweetcorn, tomatoes, mushrooms and chopped onions will all cook quickly on an already prepared pizza base. Add a sprinkling of cheese and place in the oven or under the grill for approximately 15 minutes or until the cheese is bubbling.

CARROT AND POPPY SEED MUFFINS (MAKES 12)

170 g wholemeal self-raising flour
3 eggs
2 tsps baking powder
75 g brown or muscavado sugar
1 tsp baking powder
225 g grated carrots
50 g raisins
120 ml vegetable oil
1 tsp poppy seeds (other seeds may be used instead)
Add quarter tsp nutmeg, cinnamon or ginger for flavour

Preheat the oven to 180°C/350°F/Gas mark 4. Meanwhile, mix the dry ingredients together in a large bowl, adding the carrots and raisins last. Beat the egg and oil together and then add them to the mixture, stirring the mixture until the ingredients are just combined. Spoon the mixture into greased cake moulds or cake cups and place in the oven for 20–25 minutes or until golden brown.

FRUITY OATCAKES (MAKES 12)

100 g butter
50 g date or apricot puree
100 g wholewheat flour
100 g porridge oats

Preheat the oven to 180°C/350°F/Gas mark 4. Cream the butter or margarine and fruit puree together until light. Add the flour and oats and mix to make stiff dough. Roll out the dough and cut into 12 small cakes. Bake for 15 minutes, or until lightly browned.

CRUNCHY FLAPJACKS FOR 4 PEOPLE

100 g dates
50 g fresh or dried apricots
50 g raisins or sultanas
50 g mixed pumpkin, linseed and sunflower seeds
50 g hazelnuts or walnuts
1–2 tbs lemon juice
1 tbs apple juice
110 g porridge oats

Preheat the oven to 180°C/350°F/Gas mark 4. Roughly chop all the fruit, nuts and seeds and mix with the oats and fruit juices. Press into a lightly greased baking tin and bake for approximately 15 minutes.

CHOCOLATE GRANOLA COOKIES

400 g oats
100 g barley or millet flakes (optional)
2 tbs each sunflower seeds, pumpkin seeds, sesame seeds and linseeds
200 g mixed chopped nuts or flaked almonds
50 g desiccated coconut (optional)
Honey
100 g dark chocolate

Make the granola mix as in the earlier recipe. Meanwhile, break the chocolate into chunks and melt gradually either in the microwave or in a bowl over a pan of simmering water. Keep the heat low and keep stirring the chocolate until it is just melted, then remove from the heat. Spoon cookie-sized blobs of melted chocolate onto a baking sheet and immediately sprinkle the granola mix over the chocolate. Leave it to cool and set, then carefully remove the cookies from the baking sheet.

HOME MADE COLESLAW

225 g white cabbage, grated
115 g carrots, grated
One red or white onion, chopped or sliced
1 clove of garlic, crushed or finely sliced

1 small pot fat-free Greek yoghurt
1 tbs orange juice or lemon/lime juice
1 tbs white wine vinegar

Mix the ingredients together or place in a food blender. For added omega 3 fats, add a tablespoon of linseed or rapeseed oil instead of the juice. Apple, nuts and seeds can also be added for variation.

Going organic

Three out of four households currently buy some sort of organic produce and there's no doubt that we are more interested in, and concerned about, the food that we consume. But whilst organic food may be healthier for us, is it really worth the extra time, effort and money that it may cost?

WHAT TO LOOK FOR

Any food labelled as organic must adhere to a strict set of standards – look for the Soil Association symbol (below) as a guarantee of one the highest organic standards (there are different 'levels' of organic produce).

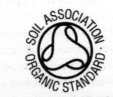

Soil Association

Any organic product sold in the UK must display the organic certification body that the food producer is registered with and a code number that ensures that UK standards have been met, although not all products will show a trademark symbol or logo.

Each EU country has its own organic certification authority with various certificating bodies. Food labelled as organic and imported from outside Europe is still subject to rigorous checks and guarantees, which also apply to all stages of food processing. However, organic products may only constitute 95 per cent of a manufactured food product with more than one ingredient added.

Farms must have achieved organic standards for two years before they gain organic status. This is to allow time for previously used pesticides, fertilizers and chemicals to be fully removed from the soil, and gives the land time to re-mineralize. However, some farms may not require this long a period for conversion.

Fish may still be considered 'organic' if it is farmed, but the conditions are different from the average fish farm, allowing more space for the fish to swim and meeting set guidelines on the use of drugs and feeding.

GOING ORGANIC – THE BENEFITS

▶ *Organic foods should have a higher nutrient content. This is because organic farmers employ crop rotation, leaving fields un-farmed for a year in between crops so that the soil can re-mineralize. As a result, organic foods will typically contain more minerals, vitamins, anti-oxidants and essential fatty acids. Some organic fruits and vegetables have also been found to contain higher levels of health-promoting phytonutrients than non-organic plants (see Chapter 3 for information on phytonutrients).*

▶ *The use of artificial chemicals and fertilizers is severely restricted so organic food will contain much lower levels* of chemicals or pesticides. Farmers can use very few pesticides on crops, which should only be used as a last resort, so although organic produce may not always be completely free of chemicals, fewer will have been used, if any at all.

▶ Organic farmers cannot grow genetically modified crops.

▶ Animals are reared without the use of antibiotics or drugs, such as growth hormones, and are fed more natural, nutritious animal feed – all this creates a healthier animal. Just as better grown plant foods are more nutritious, healthier animals and poultry also provide more nutritious meat, dairy produce and eggs containing less undesirable chemicals, such as antibiotics or growth hormones.

▶ The fatty acid ratio of eggs, milk and meat from organically reared animals and poultry is healthier than that from a non-organic source.

▶ Moral or ethical reasons for consuming organic foods are also a consideration. A strong emphasis is also placed on protecting the environment, so organic farms produce healthier food, better animal welfare and help to protect the environment.

▶ Many people find the taste of organic food vastly superior to its over-farmed equivalent. Some do not notice a difference.

▶ Although children eat less food than adults, they actually consume a higher volume of food in comparison to their body size or weight. It has been suggested that consuming large amounts of growth hormones, chemicals, fertilizers and additives from intensely farmed and processed foods may have detrimental effects upon health and development.

ARE THERE ANY DRAWBACKS?

▶ Organic food can be considerably more expensive. For example, the cost of two organic salmon fillets (£3.89) compared to the non-organic equivalent (£2.98), or organic carrots (£1.28/kg) compared with non-organic carrots (£0.68/kg) clearly shows that to 'go organic' with all of your food shopping could work out to cost substantially more than normal. However, you can always choose to consume some organic produce – it doesn't have to be 'all or nothing'.

▶ Without the additives present in non-organic produce, organic food will not last as long and may bruise more readily. It also tends to look less 'perfect' than food that has been produced to be a certain colour, shape and size.

▶ Also, as organic produce is likely to be seasonal, you may find that the variety of fruit and vegetables available is less than that stocked on supermarket shelves, although much of the inorganic produce may have been picked months earlier and stored under specific conditions to prevent it from ripening earlier.

WHERE TO FIND IT

Your local supermarket and greengrocers will have a reasonable range of organic produce, though it may cost more than the non-organic version. Local farms and box delivery services are available in most areas (though check if they are also organic) and they will deliver a selection of seasonal fruits, vegetables and other foods to your doorstep. Alternatively, friends and neighbours may grow their own produce and have some to spare or sell.

Grow your own

You could have a go at growing your own produce. Unless you have been using fertilizers, pesticides or other chemicals in your garden, the chances are that your soil should be fairly free of chemicals. However, you should check out several things to ensure that your home-grown food is good to eat:

▶ If you haven't lived at your current house for the last two years, check with the previous occupants or get a soil sample checked for mineral content.

▶ Local areas sometimes suffer with high levels of particular minerals in the soil. If one mineral is exceptionally high, this *can prevent the uptake of other minerals from the soil. A soil sample will confirm that your ground is good to sow in!*

▶ *Buy organic fertilizer or top soil to improve your own earth if you need to.*

▶ *If you haven't got a garden, contact your local council to see where the nearest allotment is and if there are spaces available.*

THINGS TO REMEMBER

Good nutrition is essential for growing children – it forms the foundations of their growing bodies and also creates many of the eating habits that they will continue throughout life. Childhood nutrition is a subject in itself, but there are some simple things you can do to help create healthy eating habits!

- *A child's fat cells are laid down during rapid growth phases – mainly during the first five years. Having more fat cells could lead to problems with weight management throughout life, so be careful not to overfeed children, especially with fatty or sugary foods, which can also create cravings.*

- *Try not to create a sweet tooth with sugary drinks and sweets. Use fruit, yoghurt, oat bars or healthy baking options as desserts and snacks from an early age.*

- *Give alternatives with no unhealthy options by asking questions like 'Do you want carrots or peas with this?' or 'Would you like a piece of apple or a slice of pear?'*

- *Have different fruits available for snacking on. This should reduce the need or craving for sugary foods. Bowls of grapes, dried apricots or strawberries are colourful and sweet to taste.*

- *Place ready-to-eat colourful vegetables at 'eye level' in the fridge so they are the first thing your child will see when they go looking for snacks. Strips of red, yellow and orange peppers, mange tout, baby corn and carrot crudités are all sweet enough to be tasty and will go down even better if they can be dipped into something like an avocado or yoghurt dip.*

- *If you are constantly snacking on chocolate, crisps or biscuits, it's more likely that your children will. Lead by example and choose a piece of fruit!*

- *Children often want foods that appear to be 'off limits' or specifically for adults ... by verbally making a fuss about how tasty specific healthy foods are, and initially telling your child that a food is 'for grown ups', this may make your child more interested in eating those foods too.*

- *Variety is the spice of life! A wide range of foods encourages children to enjoy food and experiment with different tastes. It also reduces the risk of allergies or food sensitivities forming; these can occur if specific foods are eaten too often. Eating a wide range of foods also reduces the risk of nutrient deficiencies from missing specific vitamins, minerals or fatty acids in a monotonous or processed diet.*

- *Get youngsters interested in food by helping them to create their own vegetable patch. Give them a choice (already vetted by yourself) of what they would like to grow and you could increase your family intake of healthy organic produce at a fraction of the price, whilst also finding a way to get fussy eaters to eat vegetables!*

- *Always have a jug of water on the table at meal times to encourage water consumption. A few slices of lemon or lime may make it look more enticing. Organic, fresh or pure pressed juices such as red grape, orange or apple offer a range of health benefits and 'grown up' plastic wine glasses may encourage drinking either juice or water at the dinner table.*

Taking it further

Further reading

Bourre, J. M. *Brainfood* (London: Little, Brown, 1993)

Carper, Jean, *Stop Ageing Now!* (Canada: HarperCollins/Thorson Health, 1997)

Cloutier, Marissa and Adamson, Eve, *The Mediterranean Diet* (New York: HarperCollins, 2004)

Collins Gem GL (London: HarperCollins, 2006)

Edgson, Vicki, *Food Doctor for Babies and Children* (London: Chrysalis Books, 2003)

Erasmus, Udo, *Fats that Heal, Fats that Kill* (Burnaby, BC: Alive Books, 1993)

Heber, David, *What color is your diet?* (London: HarperCollins, 2001)

Holford, Patrick, *The Optimum Nutrition Bible* (London: Piatkus, 1998)

Readers Digest, *Foods that Harm, Foods that Heal* (London: Readers Digest Association, 2007)

Simopoulos, Artemis P. and Robinson, Jo, *The Omega Diet* (London: HarperCollins, 1999)

Van Straten, Michael and Griggs, Barbara, *Superfoods* (London: Dorling Kindersley, 2006)

Useful websites

FOR NUTRITION ADVICE AND INFORMATION

The Food Standards Agency www.food.gov.uk

The British Nutrition Foundation www.nutrition.org.uk

The Food Doctor website www.thefooddoctor.com

Food and Behaviour Research www.fabresearch.org

For a list of E numbers www.ukfoodguide.net/enumeric

For information on food additives
www.foodcomm.org.uk/parentsjury

FOR INFORMATION ON ORGANIC PRODUCE AND GROWING YOUR OWN

www.directory.co.uk/Organic+Box+Deliveries.htm

www.natoora.co.uk

www.gardenorganic.org.uk

www.gardenzone.info

TO FIND A NUTRITIONAL THERAPIST IN YOUR AREA

The British Association for Nutritional Therapy
www.bant.org.uk

The Nutritional Therapy Council
www.nutritionaltherapycouncil.org.uk

FOR NUTRITIONAL SUPPLEMENTS

Archturus Healthlink Ltd. www.archturus.co.uk

Biocare www.biocare.co.uk

Nutrigold www.nutri-gold.com

The Nutri Centre (also for books) www.nutricentre.com

For nutrition information and supplements
www.nu-intelligence.com

Index

activity levels, increasing, 11–12, 50–4
additives, 237–8
ADHD, 236–7
adrenal superfoods, 199–200
adrenaline, 198, 199
ageing, 152–3
    anti-ageing diet tips, 155–68
    anti-ageing guide, 179–82
    anti-ageing nutrients, 168–72
    sun damage, 175–6
alcohol
    benefits of red wine, 167–8
    calories in, 43
    limiting intake of, 47–8, 166–7
allergies to food, 102–3, 200–5
alpha-linolenic acid (ALA), 23, 74, 132, 134, 221
aluminium theory, 241–2
Alzheimer's disease, 240–2
amino acids, 22, 97, 98, 111, 215
anaemia, 208–10
anti-carcinogenic foods, 72, 158
anti-inflammatory foods, 73–4
anti-oxidants, 61, 173, 242
    anti-ageing benefits of, 156–8
    foods rich in, 72–3, 77–8, 98, 156–8, 219

protective against free radicals, 153–5
attention deficit hyperactivity disorder (ADHD), 236–7

bacteria
    antibiotics, 206
    in probiotics, 126, 142–7
'bad' cholesterol, 137, 139, 168
'bad' fats, 159–61
basal metabolic rate (BMR), 35–6
beans
    bean casserole, 255–6
    chilli bean stew, 87–8
    mixed bean salad, 255–6
    soya beans, 75–6
berries, 72, 151, 183
beta carotene, 64, 72, 158, 170–2
blood pressure, lowering, 26
blood sugar
    conditions, 244
    controlling, 189–92
    and depression, 243
    effect of low, 229–30
body fat, 32, 75, 165
body mass index (BMI), 32–4
bones, advice for healthy, 180
books, further reading, 271
bowel health, foods for, 181
brain food, 219–20
Brazil nuts, 172

breakfasts
- detox plan, *117–21*
- for energy, *192*
- importance of, *13–14*
- omega-3 rich, *134, 162, 224, 239, 240*
- recipes, *251–3*
- for skin health, *171, 174*
- superfoods for, *80, 82–4*
- for weight loss, *55–7*

brown rice, *100*
- risotto, *254–5*

cabbage, *71*
- coleslaw, *263–4*
- savoy cabbage stir fry, *86*

caffeine
- effects of, *197–8*
- giving up, *109–10*
- and insomnia, *210–11*

calorie-saving chart, *44–5*

calories
- in certain foods, *42–3*
- exercising to use up, *50–4*
- reducing intake of, *40–50*
- restricting to stay young, *155–6*

candidiasis, *205–8*

carbohydrates, *6, 20–1*
- amount to eat, *193*
- reducing intake of refined, *164–5*

carotene, *64, 72, 158, 170–2, 183*

carotenoids, *63–4, 140*
- beta carotene, *72, 158, 170–2*
- lutein, *71*
- lycopene, *71–2*

carrots and poppy seed muffins, *262*

catechins, *63, 77*

cherries, *72*

children
- brain foods, *238–9*
- effect of additives on, *237–8*
- healthy recipes for, *261–4*
- hyperactivity, *236–7*
- involving in cooking, *260*

chilli bean stew, *87–8*

chocolate, *216*
- best type of, *217–18*
- cravings for, *191, 218*
- granola cookies, *263*
- mineral content in, *219*
- stimulant qualities, *216–17*

cholesterol-lowering foods, *26–7, 65–6, 138–40*

chronic fatigue syndrome, *211–12*

citrus fruits, benefits of, *183*

Co-enzyme A, *194*

cod liver oil, *222*

coeliac disease, *204*

coffee
- alternatives to, *65, 109*
- effects of drinking, *197–8*

colds and coughs, *114*

coleslaw, *263–4*

collagen, *173*

complete protein, *22, 23*

complex carbohydrates, *21*

constipation, *114*

coronary heart disease, reducing risk of, *26–7*

cruciferous vegetables, *71, 158*

curry, superfood recipe, *84–5*
cyclic food allergies, *202*
cystitis, *114*

dairy food allergies, *204*
dehydration, *12, 195–6*
    face mask for dehydrated
      skin, *177*
dementia, *239–40, 242*
depression, *242–3*
detoxification, *92–3*
    14 day detox plan, *117–21*
    basic guidelines, *108–10*
    the detox plan, *115–16*
    different levels of, *101–4*
    need for, *95–6*
    options, *100–1*
    phases of, *97–100*
    planning, *104–7*
    possible side effects,
      113–15
    reasons for, *93–5*
    supplements to help,
      110–12
    top 10 foods for, *107–8*
    toxins, *96–7*
    what to expect during,
      112–13
diabetes, *191*
    benefits of green tea, *77*
    foods reducing risk of,
      180, 192
    and sugar intake, *164–5*
diarrhoea, *111–12, 114*
dietary advice, sources of, *4–5*
digestive health, foods for, *181*
dinners
    20-minute meals, *257–8*

detox plan, *117–21*
    for energy, *192*
    omega 3 rich, *134, 162,
      224, 240*
    recipes, *254–7*
    for skin health, *172, 174*
    superfoods, *81, 82–4*
    for weight loss, *55–7*
disaccharides, *21*
docosahexanoic acid (DHA),
    73–4, 220, 222, 241, 246
dysbiosis, *143–4, 206–7*

eating out, *46–7*
eggs, omega 3 enriched, *133,
    135–7*
eicosapentanoic acid (EPA),
    73–4, 220, 222, 246
elimination, *99–100*
endotoxins, *96*
energy, *185–6*
    adrenal superfoods,
      199–200
    allergies, *200–5*
    anaemia, *208–10*
    blood sugar control,
      189–92
    caffeinated drinks, *197–8*
    candidiasis, *205–8*
    carbohydrate requirements,
      193
    chronic fatigue syndrome,
      211–12
    dehydration, *195–6*
    energy balance equation,
      30–2
    energy giving foods, *193–5*
    fluid intake, *196–7*

glycaemic index/load, 187–9
  insomnia, 210–11
  stress, 199
energy balance equation, 30–2
enzyme-inducers, 61
essential amino acids, 22–3, 215, 234
essential fatty acids, 24, 66–9, 73–4, 162–3, 236–7
evening primrose oil, 236
exercise, 11–12
  and energy balance, 31
  extra calories for, 36
  for weight loss, 50–4
exotoxins, 96
eye health, foods for, 181–2

family involvement, 260–70
fasting hypoglycaemia, 244
fats, 23–5
  'bad' fats, 159–61
  'good' fats, 161–3
  and oxidation, 163–4
fibre, 25–6
fish, 73–4
  alternatives to, 68, 74, 132, 220–1
  and Alzheimer's disease, 241
  menu ideas, 162, 240
  organically farmed, 137
  recipes, 85, 86–7, 88–9, 175, 258
  recommended intake, 8–9
  time-saving tips, 259
  see also oily fish
fish oil supplements, 73, 132

'five a day' advice, 7–8
flapjacks, 263
flavonoids, 62–3, 69
flaxseed (linseed), 74, 221
fluid intake, increasing, 196–7
folic acid, 226, 228
food allergies, 200–5
food diaries, 2–4, 41
food groups, 5–6
free radicals, 98, 153–5
  limiting damage due to, 164
French paradox, 167
fruit, 71–3
  and Alzheimer's disease, 241, 242
  'five a day', 7–8
  fruit salad, 251
  health benefits of, 26–7, 142
functional foods, 123–5
  benefits and drawbacks of, 128–30
  cost of, 141–2
  deciding what's best, 147–9
  omega 3 fatty acids, 130–7
  plant sterols, 137–40
  probiotic and prebiotic revolution, 142–7
  problems with, 125
  usefulness of, 127–8

garlic, 70–1, 179, 184
Gingko biloba, 245
glucose levels, 165–6, 189–92
  effect of chocolate, 216
  see also blood sugar
gluten, allergy to, 204

glycaemic index (GI), 21, 187–9
glycaemic load (GL), 187–9
'good' cholesterol, 136, 168
'good' fats, 161–3
government tips for a healthy diet, 6
grains, see brown rice; oats
granola recipe, 252
grape seeds, 73
grapes, red, 72, 184
green leafy vegetables, 71, 78–9, 183
green tea, 76–7, 110, 158, 183
growing your own food, 267–8

hair, nutrition for healthy, 177–8
HDL (high-density lipoprotein), see 'good' cholesterol
headaches, 115
healthy diet, 2
    and improved health, 26–7
    recommendations, 4–14
heart disease
    and alcohol, 166–8
    and essential fatty acids, 67–8
    reducing risk of, 26–7, 179–80
herbal teas, 109–10
herbs, 79–80
high-protein diets, 192
hydrogenated fats, 138, 160
hyperactivity, 236–8
hypoglycaemia, 234, 244

immune function, foods for, 180–1
incomplete protein, 22

insoluble fibre, 25
insomnia, 210–11
insulin, 164–5, 190, 198
interval training, 54
inulin, 66, 70, 147
iron deficiency, 208–10
isoflavones, beans, 63, 75–6
isoflavonoids, citrus fruit, 63

joint health, foods for, 180
juices, 134, 241
junk foods vs. whole foods, 237

kedgeree, 85
kidneys
    food for healthy, 178
    function of, 100

LDL (low-density lipoprotein), see 'bad' cholesterol
lecithin (phosphatidyl choline), 110–11
legislation, 125
lifestyle changes, 19–20, 250–1
linoleic acid, see omega 6 fatty acids
linolenic acid (LNA), see omega 3 fatty acids
linseeds/linseed oil, 74, 221
liver, detox role of, 94, 97
long chain fatty acids, 68, 73, 220, 236–7, 240, 241
longevity, see ageing
low blood sugar levels, 229, 243–4
lunches
    brain boosting, 239
    detox plan, 117–21
    for energy, 192

omega 3-rich, *162, 224, 239, 240*
for skin health, *171, 174*
superfoods for, *81, 82–4*
time-saving ideas, *254–7*
tuck box ideas, *253–4*
for weight loss, *55–7*
lutein, *64, 71*
lycopene, *64, 71–2*

magnesium-rich foods, *78, 218*
margarines, *126*
enriched, *127, 134, 138–9*
hydrogenated fats in, *160*
masked food allergies, *203*
Mediterranean-style diet, *9, 27, 139, 161*
Mediterranean-style salad, *257*
mental function, increasing, *181, 244–6*
mental health conditions, *230*
ADHD, *236–9*
Alzheimer's disease, *240–2*
dementia, *239–40*
depression, *242–4*
insomnia, *230–3*
pre-menstrual tension (PMT), *233–6*
milk chocolate, *218*
milk thistle (Silymarin), *110*
mineral supplements, *111, 228*
monosaccharides, *21*
monounsaturated fats, *24–5, 161*
mood diaries, *243, 244*
mood swings, *230*
muesli recipe, *252*
myalgic encephalitis (ME), *211–12*

nails, nutrition for, *178–9*
niacin, *194, 225–6*
nutrition in foods, maximizing, *89*
nutrition quiz, *16–19*
nuts, *66, 74, 170, 172, 184, 195*

oats, *66*
granola, *252*
porridge, *252–3*
recipes using, *262–3*
oils
omega 3 content, *74, 221*
oxidation of, *163–4*
oily fish, *8–9, 73–4, 183, 223*
and brain function, *68, 219–20*
see also fish
olive oil, *161, 221*
omega 3 fatty acids, *23–4, 131–2*
conditions needing more, *131*
in eggs, *135–6*
fish oil supplements, *73, 132*
foods naturally containing, *131, 221*
in functional foods, *130, 132*
for healthy hair, *177*
in nuts, seeds and oils, *74*
in oily fish, *8–9, 73, 219–20*
and omega 6 ratio, *66–7, 130*
and PMT, *234–5, 236*

omega 6 fatty acids, *23, 24, 66, 68*
   excess consumption of, *67, 75, 130*
   in nuts, seeds and oils, *74*
onions, *69*
optimum nutrition, *14–20*
ORAC (Oxygen Radical Absorbance Capacity, *157*
organic foods, *264–8*
oxidative damage, *163–4*

pantothenic acid, *194, 195*
phosphatidyl serine, *245–6*
phyto-oestrogens, *76*
phytonutrients, *61–6*
phytosterols, *65, 126, 129, 137–40*
pizza, *261–2*
plant sterols, *137–40*
polyphenols in red wine, *168*
polysaccharides, *21*
polyunsaturated fats, *25, 161*
porridge, *252–3*
portion sizes, *7–8, 48–50*
potassium, sources of, *78, 178*
potatoes
   baked potato dinner, *255*
   potato salads, *255, 257*
   sweet potato recipes, *86–7, 175*
pre-menstrual tension (PMT), *218, 233–6*
prebiotics, *142–3, 147*
priorities, deciding, *15*
proanthocyanidins, *63, 72–3, 184*
probiotics, *142–7*

protein, *21–3*
   high-protein diets, *192*
   protein glycosylation, *165–6*
psyllium husk powder, *111–12*

rapeseed oil, *221*
reactive hypoglycaemia, *244*
recipes
   breakfast ideas, *251–3*
   superfood, *84–9*
   time saving, *254–8*
   for tuck boxes, *253–4*
   for young cooks, *261–4*
red bush tea, *110*
red wine, *72, 167–8, 184*
rice, brown, *100*
   recipes, *254–5*
Rooibosch (red bush) tea, *110*

salad leaves, nutrients in, *78–9*
salads
   anti-oxidant fix, *156–7*
   mediterranean-style, *257*
   rice salad, *254–5*
   time-saving tips, *259*
salmon
   parcels, *258*
   and stir fry vegetables, *88–9*
   and sweet potato risotto, *86–7, 175*
salt, cutting back on, *10–11, 178*
saturated fats, *24*
   reducing, *9, 159*
savoy cabbage stir fry, *86*

seeds/seed oils, *75, 184*
    omega 3 content, *74*
selenium, *172*
serotonin, *215–16, 234*
shopping, *47*
    for carotenoids, *64*
    for detox diet, *106–7*
    store cupboard basics, *81–2*
simple carbohydrates, *21*
skin conditions, *114–15*
skin health
    beta carotene, *171*
    face masks, *77, 177*
    nutrition for, *173–6, 179*
    water, *176*
sleep problems, *210–11*
SMART goals for weight loss, *38–40*
sodium content in foods, *10–11*
Soil Association, *264*
soluble fibre, *25*
soup
    time-saving tips, *258–9*
    vegetable, *256–7*
soya/soya beans, *75–6, 184*
spices, *79–80*
spots, *114–15*
St. John's Wort, *245*
starchy foods, *6, 193*
stir fry, *86, 88–9, 257*
store cupboard basics, *81–2*
stress, *199, 206*
sugar, cutting down on, *10, 164–6*
sulphur compounds, *64–5*
sun damage, *175–6*

superfoods, *60–1*
    7-day eating plan, *82–4*
    for adrenal glands, *199–200*
    berries, cherries and grapes, *72–3*
    brassicas, *71*
    carotene-rich foods, *72*
    essential fatty acids, *66–9*
    garlic, *70–1*
    getting the most from, *89–90*
    green tea, *76–7*
    oily fish, *73–4*
    onions, *69*
    phytonutrients, *61–6*
    recipes, *84–9*
    seeds/seed oils, *75*
    soya beans, *75–6*
    tomatoes, *71–2*
    turmeric, *77–8*
supplements, *110–12*
    cod liver oil, *222*
    nutrients, *228*
    to help mental function, *244–6*
sweet potato, *86–7, 175*

tea
    green tea, *76–7, 110, 158, 183*
    herbal teas, *109–10*
thiamine, *194, 225*
thrush, *206, 208*
tomato soup, *85–6*
tomatoes, *71–2*
tortilla wraps, *254*
toxins, *96–7, 99*
trans fats, *138, 160–1*

tryptophan, *215, 232–3*
tuck box ideas, *253–4*
tuna
    seared tuna steak, *87*
    tinned, *9, 220*
turmeric, *77–8*

vegetables, *71*
    and Alzheimer's disease, *241*
    'five a day' advice, *7–8*
    health benefits of, *26–7, 142*
    pizza recipe, *261–2*
    stuffed baked, *88*
    time-saving tips, *259*
    vegetable proteins, *23*
    vegetable stew, *256–7*
vegetarians
    iron-rich foods, *209, 232*
    omega 3 menu, *162*
    protein for, *23*
vitamins
    fat soluble, *24*
    and PMT, *235*
    in salad leaves, *79*
    supplements, *111*
    for vitality, *199–200*
    vitamin B, *194–5, 200, 225–7, 228–9*
    vitamin C, *79, 169, 183, 194, 200, 209*
    vitamin E, *169–70, 172, 173*

water, *12–13, 184*
    and dehydration, *195–6*
    for eliminating toxins, *100*

hot water during a detox, *108–9*
increasing intake of, *176, 196–7*
water-soluble compounds/ toxins, *98–9*
websites, *272–3*
weight-bearing exercise, *53*
weight control
    7 day eating plan, *55–7*
    basal metabolic rate (BMR), *35–6*
    body mass index (BMI), *32–4*
    calculating how much to lose, *36–7*
    eating less and exercising more, *54–5*
    energy balance equation, *30–2*
    from exercising, *50–4*
    reasons for weight gain, *29–30*
    reducing calorie intake, *40–50*
    setting goals, *37–40*
weight training, *54*
wheat allergy, *102–3, 202, 203, 204*
white fish, *74, 223*
whole foods vs. junk foods, *237*
wine, benefits of red, *72, 167–8*

yeast infections, *205–8*
yoghurts/yoghurt drinks, *126*

zinc, *179, 227, 228, 233*

Image credits